MW01178863

Massage

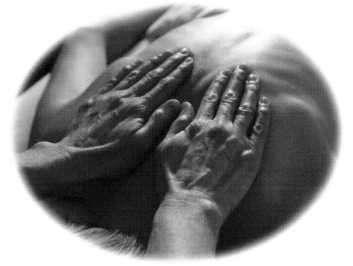

Written by Mike Dowling

TOP THAT!™

Copyright © 2004 Top That! Publishing Inc,
25031 W. Avenue Stanford, Suite #60, Valencia, CA 91355
All rights reserved
www.topthatpublishing.com

CONTENTS

List of ingredients for the carrier and essential oils
contained in this pack:
Carrier Oil
Ingredients: Canola Oil, Tocopherol Acetate (Vit. E).

Lavender
Ingredients: Mineral Oil, Jojoba Oil, Lavender Oil,
Tocopherol Acetate (Vit. E),
T-Butyl Hydroquinone.

Ylang Ylang
Ingredients: Mineral Oil, Jojoba Oil, Ylang Ylang Oil,
Tocopherol Acetate (Vit. E),
T-Butyl Hydroquinone.

Geranium
Ingredients: Mineral Oil, Jojoba Oil,
Geranium Oil, Tocopherol Acetate (Vit. E),
T-Butyl Hydroquinone.

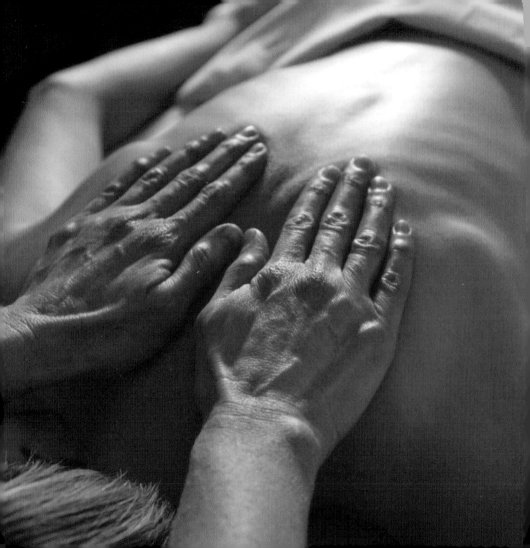

INTRODUCTION

MASSAGE IS PROBABLY THE OLDEST FORM OF HEALING.
EVERY DAY WE USE TOUCH INSTINCTIVELY TO HELP SOOTHE
AND COMFORT OURSELVES AND OTHERS.

In the animal kingdom young creatures snuggle up to each other for warmth and comfort. Primates pat and lay hands on each other for reassurance, and social grooming is part of normal everyday behavior.

The Chinese had a system of massage about five thousand years ago. Four thousand years ago the Hindu culture referred to massage as "rubbing and shampooing" and other references occur in Egyptian, Persian, and Japanese literature. Hippocrates, the ancient Greek regarded as the father of medicine, wrote: "A physician must be experienced in many things but assuredly in rubbing."

WARNING:

THE OILS CONTAINED IN THIS PACK ARE CONCENTRATED
MATERIALS AND MUST BE DILUTED WITH A CARRIER OIL.
DO NOT INGEST, IF INGESTED DO NOT INDUCE VOMITING
AND SEEK MEDICAL ATTENTION IMMEDIATELY. KEEP OUT OF
THE REACH OF CHILDREN. AVOID CONTACT WITH EYES, RINSE
THOROUGHLY WITH WARM WATER IF THIS OCCURS. PRIOR TO
USE CHECK FOR SKIN SENSITIVITY USING A PATCH TEST,
DISCONTINUE USE IF ANY ADVERSE REACTIONS OCCUR.

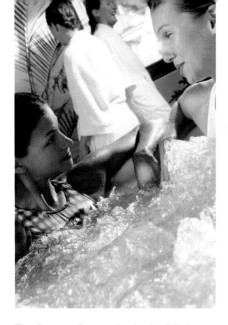

The famous Roman baths had little to do with water. The bathing process consisted of a massage in a sweet-smelling oil, which was then scraped off using the equivalent of a blunt razor.

The oil cleansed by absorbing dirt and grime and the water was only used as a rinse afterwards.

At the beginning of the nineteenth century, a Swedish man called Pehr Henrik Ling studied different forms of massage and traveled to China to experience the methods there. He set up his own system and classified movements that later became known as Swedish massage. The system he created is still the basis of most osteopathic and orthopedic diagnosis today.

In recent years there has been a considerable revival of interest in massage as both a therapy and a general recreational activity. This book is an introduction to the subject and will help you to learn basic movements that you can try safely and enjoy.

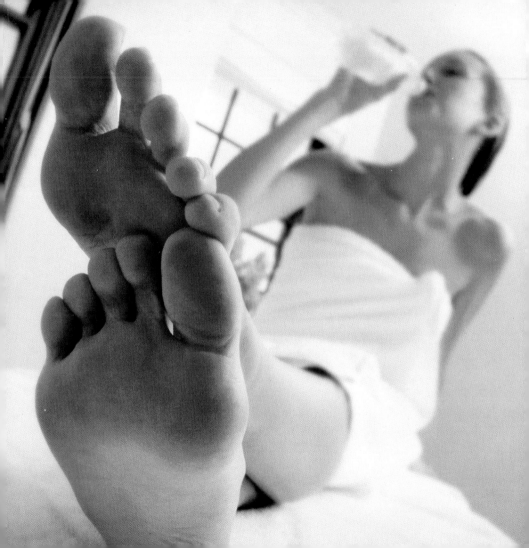

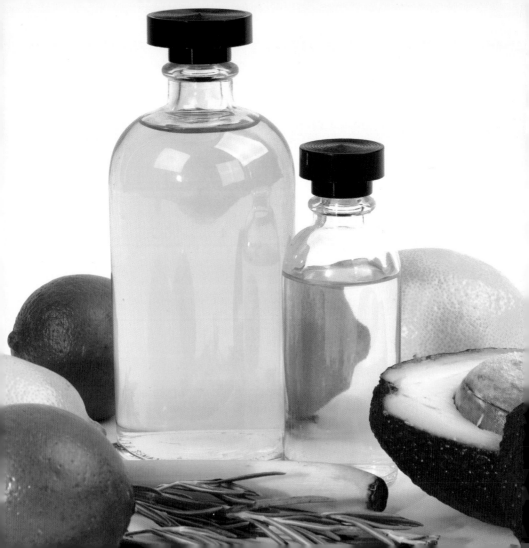

CARRIER OILS

ESSENTIAL OILS ARE VERY STRONG. IF YOU
WANT TO USE THEM FOR MASSAGE THEY
MUST BE DILUTED WITH A CARRIER OIL.

Carrier oils are so called because they are used to "carry" the various essential oils that are beneficial in massage.

Often it is the therapeutic properties of the essential oils that are being sought in a massage, but the high concentrations of these oils on their own make some of them potentially dangerous to use directly on the skin. It is important, therefore, to mix essential oils with a carrier oil to make them safe to use in massage.

Unlike essential oils, carrier oils do not evaporate when they are heated and so are sometimes called "fixed oils." In massage, carrier oils are also known as base oils.

While they vary greatly in price do not be tempted to compromise. Always try to get "cold-pressed" oils, sometimes called "extra virgin," from a reputable supplier. Which oil you decide to use is really down to personal preference. Some have a distinct fragrance of their own, while others are quite bland. Peach and apricot kernel are both good carrier oils.

Carrier oils tend to last about three months before they go rancid. Adding ten per cent of wheatgerm oil will make your mixtures last twice as long. You can usually buy small quantities of carrier oils so that you do not waste them. Keep your bottles as full as possible to eliminate air and store them in a cool, dark place.

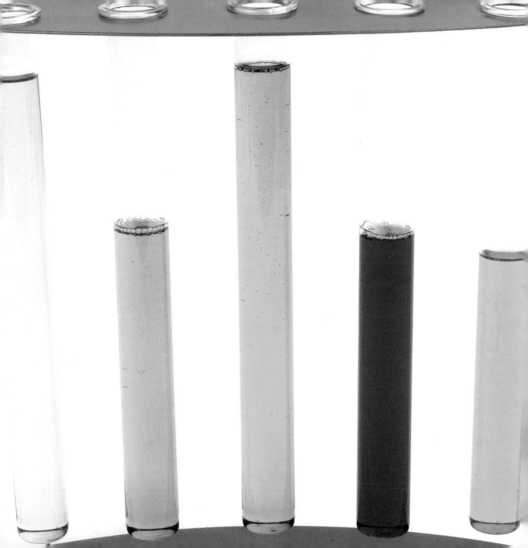

BLENDING OILS

YOU CAN BUY READY-MADE MASSAGE OILS BUT THEY CAN BE EXPENSIVE AND IT IS EASY, AND ENJOYABLE, TO MAKE YOUR OWN.

The base, or carrier, oil should be a natural, cold-pressed vegetable oil of which there are quite a selection.

Almond oil is comparatively inexpensive and has the benefit of little, if any, scent of its own, making it ideal for the addition of essential oils. It is also slightly adhesive which makes it a little less slippery than some oils during massage.

Apricot and peach kernel are lovely oils and smell slightly of their respective fruits. Jojoba, which is actually a liquid wax, is wonderful on the skin. These three are somewhat expensive but provide beautifully extravagant bases!

When mixing your oils, a plastic flip-top bottle is ideal but you can just as easily use a cup or suitable bowl. Make sure that you have somewhere safe to stand them, as you don't want to knock them over during the massage.

Blending oils is something of an art but practice makes perfect!

For use on the skin, as an addition to massage oil, it is vital that essential oils are diluted. This will usually be done in a vegetable oil although creams can be used as well.

The concentration of essential oils when mixed for adults should not

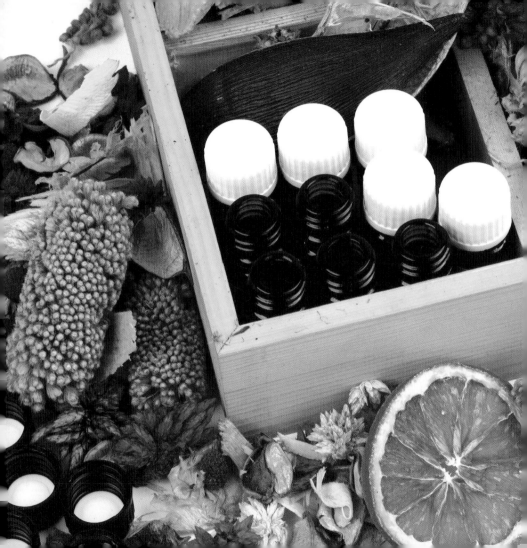

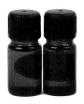

exceed two and a half per cent and, for children under fourteen, one per cent. This sounds complicated but is quite simple to work out. The size of a drop from a standard essential oil bottle is remarkably uniform. One hundred drops of oil equals one teaspoon (1 tsp). So, for a one per cent dilution you would use one drop of essential oil per teaspoon of carrier and for a two per cent dilution, two drops.

A teaspoonful is enough for a face massage and a full body massage takes about five teaspoonfuls so you should just add drops of essential oils accordingly.

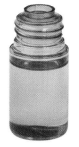

WARNING:

SOME INDIVIDUALS MAY BE PARTICULARLY SENSITIVE TO CERTAIN OILS. BEFORE USING ANY NEW OR UNFAMILIAR OILS, INCLUDING THOSE PROVIDED IN THIS BOX SET, IT IS ADVISABLE TO CONDUCT A PATCH TEST. APPLY A SMALL AMOUNT OF APPROPRIATELY MIXED OIL TO THE INSIDE OF THE RECIPIENT'S ARM. LEAVE FOR 24 HOURS AND DISCONTINUE USE IF ANY ADVERSE REACTION OCCURS.
THE OILS CONTAINED IN THIS PACK ARE NOT SUITABLE FOR USE ON INFANTS OR CHILDREN.

MIXING OILS

THERE ARE A NUMBER OF SUGGESTED BLENDS SERVING DIFFERENT PURPOSES.

Essential oils can be combined to impart their therapeutic effects during massage. They do, however, only keep for around three months when mixed with a base oil and should be discarded thereafter.

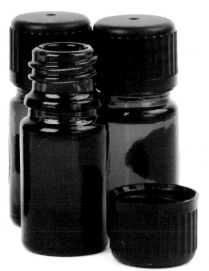

AN INVIGORATING MASSAGE OIL

7 drops rosewood

3 drops orange

2 drops geranium in 5 tsp base oil

OIL FOR MATURE PEOPLE

4 drops frankincense

4 drops cypress

4 drops lavender in 5 tsp base oil

OIL FOR YOUNG PEOPLE

5 drops mandarin

5 drops lavender

2 drops geranium in 5 tsp base oil

OIL FOR DRY SKIN

5 drops sandalwood

3 drops geranium

2 drops rosewood

2 drops ylang ylang in 5 tsp base oil

OIL FOR OILY SKIN

6 drops cypress

6 drops lemon in 5 tsp base oil

OIL FOR INFLAMED OR SENSITIVE SKIN

2 drops Roman chamomile

2 drops rose

2 drops neroli in 5 tsp base oil

FOR COLDS AND SINUS PROBLEMS

3 drops marjoram

6 drops eucalyptus

3 drops peppermint in 5 tsp base oil

Not suitable for children

FOR HEADACHES

5 drops lavender

or rosemary in 5 tsp base oil

FOR MUSCULAR ACHES

5 drops juniper

4 drops lavender

3 drops rosemary in 5 tsp base oil

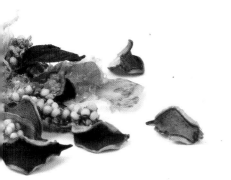
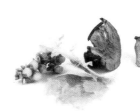
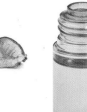

A SENSUAL MASSAGE OIL

2 drops jasmine

2 drops rose

5 drops sandalwood

2 drops bergamot in 5 tsp base oil

A RELAXING MASSAGE OIL

6 drops lavender

2 drops geranium

6 drops sandalwood in 5 tsp base oil

A "SLOW DOWN" RECIPE

4 drops marjoram

4 drops frankincense

4 drops neroli in 5 tsp base oil

A "CHEER UP" RECIPE

4 drops clary sage

4 drops bergamot

4 drops ylang ylang in 5 tsp base oil

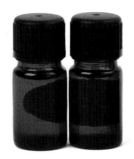

Alternatively, you could try out the lavender, geranium, and ylang ylang oils that are included in this pack.

Although ready-mixed with jojoba oil, all three oils still need to be diluted with a suitable amount of carrier oil before use.

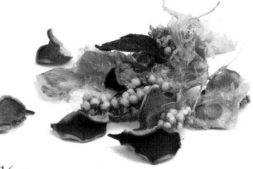

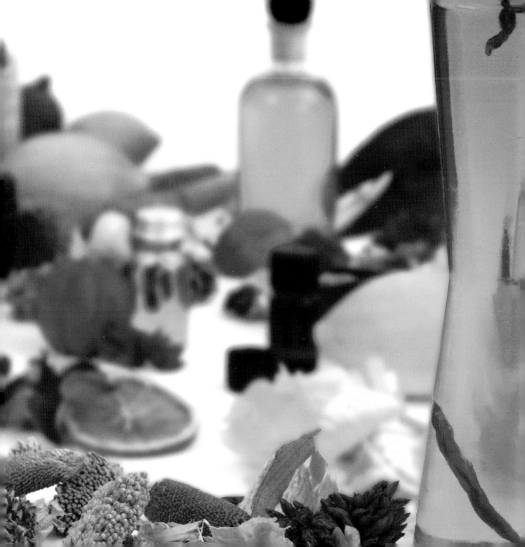

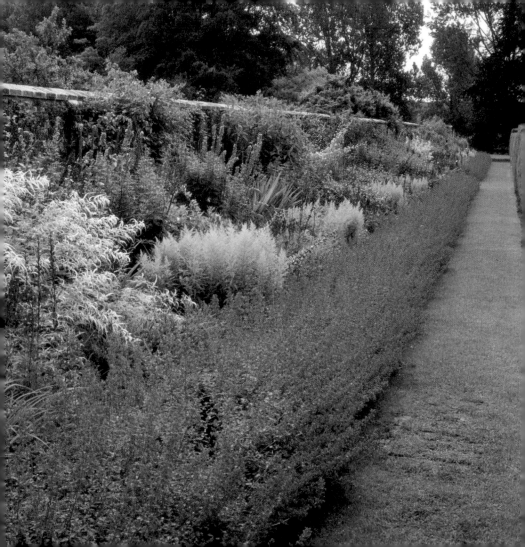

LAVENDER

Lavandula Angustifolium

A COLORLESS OIL WITH A SWEET, WOODY, AND FLORAL SCENT. THIS IS PROBABLY THE MOST FAMILIAR MASSAGE OIL AND CERTAINLY THE MOST POPULAR.

Unfortunately, lavender's popularity has made it quite difficult to obtain good-quality, unadulterated oil but it certainly is the one that every home should have.

As an essential oil, it has so many uses that a full list is practically impossible.

Its healing properties are remarkable as it accelerates cell growth and repair. It is a sedative and analgesic, and helps with high blood pressure, rheumatic pain, and muscular aches.

Use it with a carrier oil to help dermatitis, dry eczema, acne, headaches, depression, insomnia, migraine, and bruises.

If you run out of things to try it on, it is even said to be an antidote to black widow spider venom!

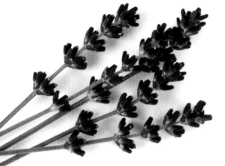

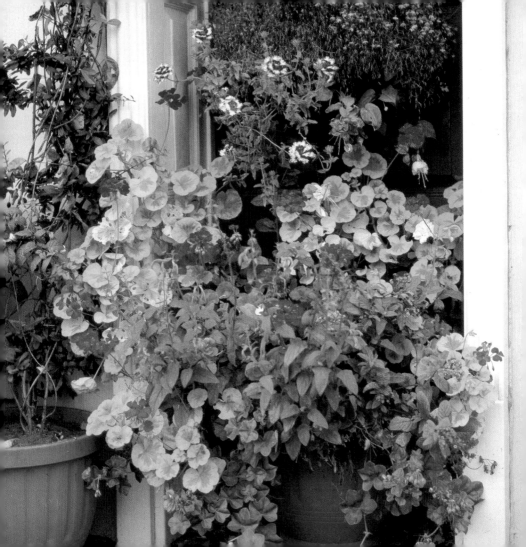

GERANIUM

Pelargonium Odaratissimum

A GREEN-COLORED OIL WITH A HEAVY, ROSY SCENT.
IT IS SAID TO BE BALANCING AND HARMONIZING AND HELPS
THE BODY TO WORK WELL AS A UNIT.

Geranium oil contains estrogenic substances which can assist with PMS and menstrual problems.

It is a gentle analgesic and antiseptic. Skin problems including dry skin, acne, and dry eczema will also benefit from this oil's properties. A good insect repellent, it is also a useful oil for people who experience mood swings.

It blends well with many essential oils which should then be diluted with a carrier oil.

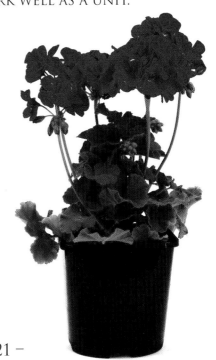

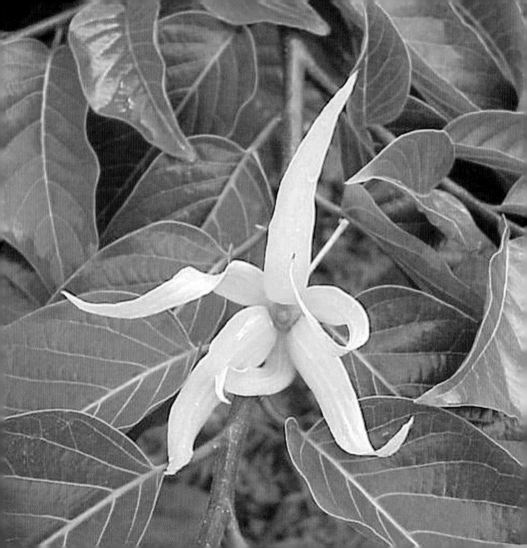

YLANG YLANG

Cananga Odorata

THIS IS A PALE YELLOW OIL WITH A VERY SWEET, HEADY, FLORAL AROMA. IT IS SOMETIMES CALLED "POOR MAN'S JASMINE."

Ylang ylang oil has a reputation as an aphrodisiac and is recommended for impotence or frigidity.

Its sedative properties make it useful for anxiety and stress conditions as it slows the breathing and heart rate.

Certain skin conditions, particularly acne or oily skin, can respond to this oil since it helps to balance sebum.

However, beware, ylang ylang is a very powerful fragrance and should be used sparingly as too much can give you a headache. Blending with a carrier oil is necessary, and should also help to combat the heady scent.

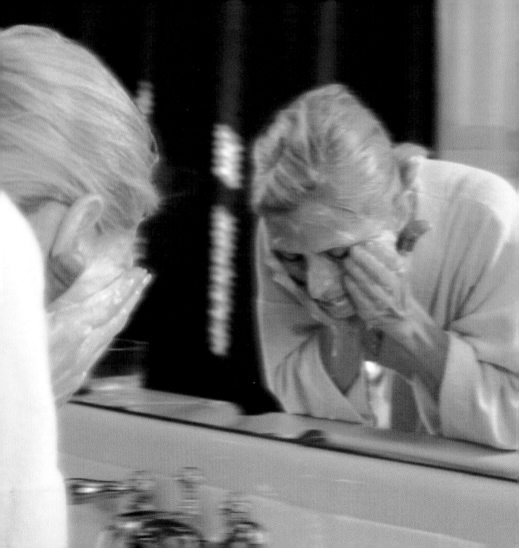

JOJOBA
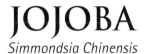
Simmondsia Chinensis

JOJOBA IS NOT AN OIL BUT, IN FACT, A LIQUID WAX
EXTRACTED FROM THE BEANS OF THE PLANT.

Jojoba becomes quite solid at cool temperatures and is pale yellow in color. Its chemical composition is very similar to that of skin sebum and its anti-bacterial properties give it a long shelf-life.

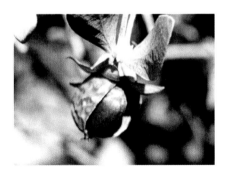

Used extensively in the beauty industry, it is valuable on all types of skin as a cleanser and a "wrinkle fighter!"

It re-hydrates mature skin and is valuable in treating psoriasis and eczema. Commonly found in many commercial shampoos, it is wonderful for hair.

It is also thought to have some anti-inflammatory properties.

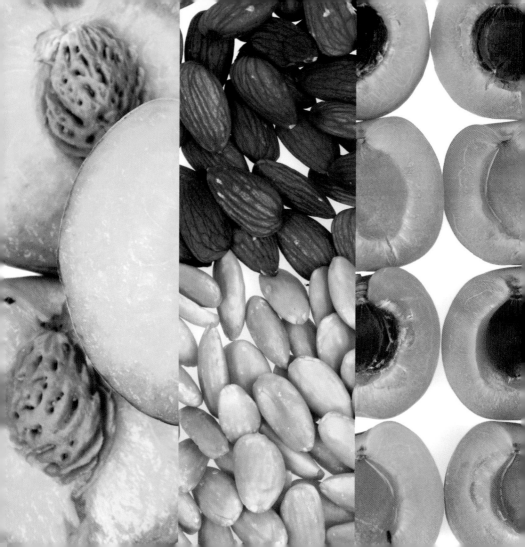

OTHER OILS AVAILABLE

APRICOT, PEACH, AND SWEET ALMOND
ALL MAKE EXCELLENT CARRIER OILS AND
SHOULD BE INCLUDED IN YOUR COLLECTION.

APRICOT *Prunus Armeniaca*
A lovely, light, pale yellow oil which has a slight smell of marzipan. It is very easily absorbed into the surface of the skin. It contains vitamins A and C and is suitable for all types of skin, but especially prematurely aged, inflamed, dry, or sensitive skin. It can help relieve itching and makes a lovely base for a face or body massage.

PEACH *Prunus Persica*
This is a luxurious carrier oil with a smooth texture, golden color and faint peach aroma. It is quite expensive and is extracted by expression from the kernels. It is a wonderful base oil for facial massage as it encourages the skin to secrete its own natural oils and prevent dehydration. It keeps the skin supple and elastic and is very good for sensitive complexions. It can be mixed easily with other base oils.

SWEET ALMOND *Prunus Dulcis*
This carrier oil is probably the most popular base oil for massage use. It is extracted by expression to give a pale yellow, fairly light, nearly odorless oil, ideal for the addition of essential oils. Containing a number of vitamins, it is very nourishing for dry skin. Anti-inflammatory properties make it valuable for psoriasis, eczema, and dermatitis. Make the effort to find a good source of this oil as sometimes it is obtained using a heating process which destroys the vitamins and nutritional qualities.

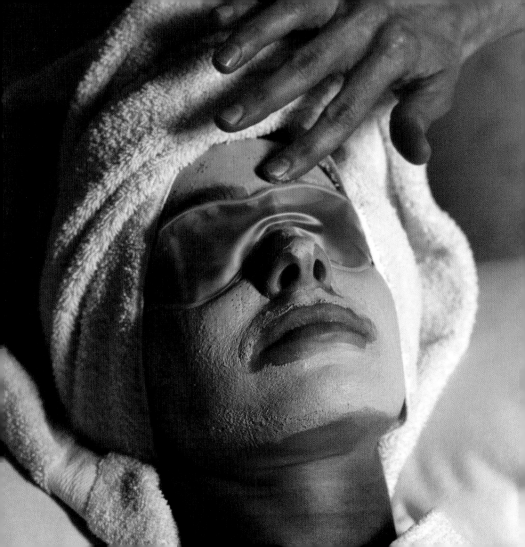

BENEFITS OF MASSAGE

MASSAGE IS A METHOD OF MANIPULATING THE SOFT
TISSUES OF THE BODY. ITS MAIN OBJECTIVES ARE
RELAXATION AND THE RESTORATION OF FUNCTION.

✓ It is invaluable where blood circulation is restricted or sluggish, or when the lymphatic system has been compromised through illness or disease.

✓ Massage aids skin health and thus the elimination of toxins from the body. The removal of waste products in the muscular system that can lead to tension and immobility can be assisted by massage. It can also help with the breakdown and removal of fat deposits in the body.

✓ It provides a form of passive exercise, whereby the muscles contract and relax without the individual having to do anything themselves. By stimulating the nervous system and increasing cellular metabolism, it can relieve pain, loosen scar tissue, and stretch adhesions.

✓ Perhaps the most important benefit of massage is that of bringing relaxation to the recipient. It offers a little time to feel pampered and an opportunity for the body to take a break and unwind.

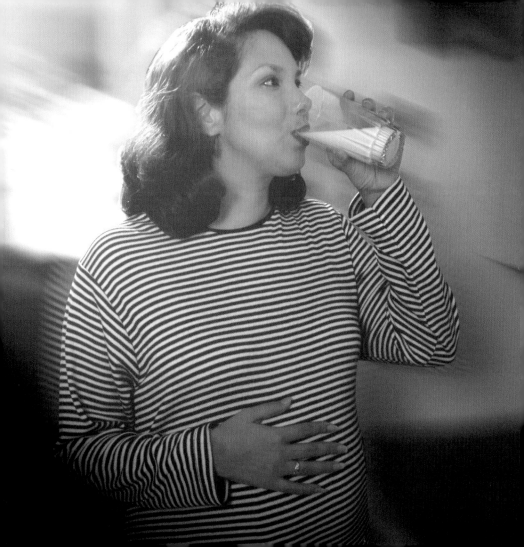

SAFETY TIPS

THERE ARE SITUATIONS WHERE MASSAGE SHOULD BE
AVOIDED AND ALTHOUGH REALLY A MATTER OF COMMON
SENSE, IT IS STILL WORTH MENTIONING A FEW.

✗ Massage should never be used over areas with varicose veins, as there is serious danger they could rupture or move blood clots into more hazardous areas of the body.

✗ It is unwise to massage over the abdomen during the first three months of pregnancy, or over recent scar tissue.

✗ Do not massage over unrecognized lumps or bumps, septic areas, or damaged skin. Inflamed areas should also be avoided.

✗ People suffering from epilepsy, diabetes, or any other medical condition should only be treated by a professional massage therapist, after consultation with a doctor.

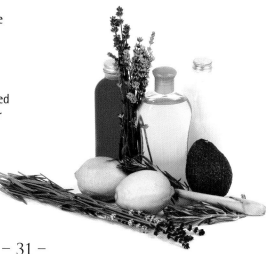

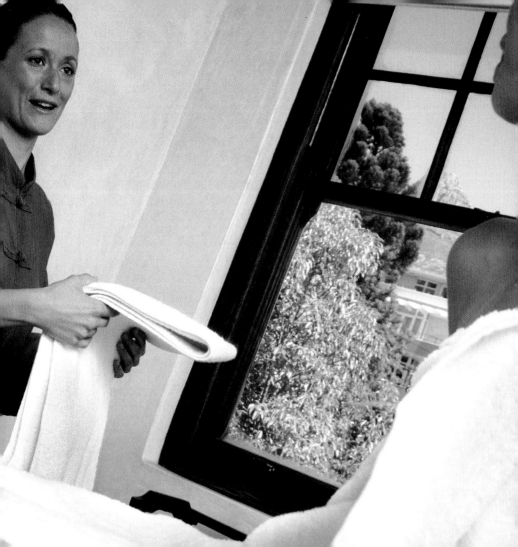

REQUIREMENTS

MASSAGE CAN BE DONE ALMOST ANYWHERE AND, IN ITS MOST BASIC FORM, AT ANY TIME.

A head, neck, or foot massage can be done with the recipient sitting in a chair. For a proper full-body massage, a traditional massage table is undoubtedly best but they can be expensive and awkward to accommodate.

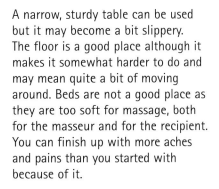

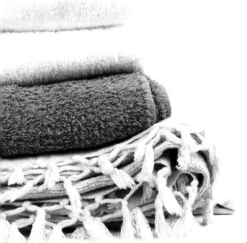

A narrow, sturdy table can be used but it may become a bit slippery. The floor is a good place although it makes it somewhat harder to do and may mean quite a bit of moving around. Beds are not a good place as they are too soft for massage, both for the masseur and for the recipient. You can finish up with more aches and pains than you started with because of it.

Assuming that the recipient is going to be lying down, you will need some sort of padding for them to lie on. A foam pad between one and two inches thick works well. If this is not possible, a couple of sleeping bags, blankets, or a duvet will do.

Alternatively, you could place a single mattress directly on the floor. Whatever padding you use, it is a good idea to cover it with a plastic sheet and then a bed sheet on top. This will prevent oil getting onto the padding, clothes, or carpets. Oil can stain and is difficult to wash out.

The best massage medium is a good-quality vegetable oil, which will provide vitamins and minerals for the skin.

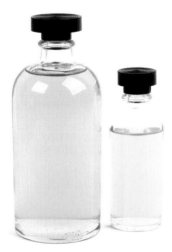

It will be absorbed into the top layers of the skin while providing some lubrication for the masseur's hands. Used sparingly, it also gives a little adhesion and makes the massage strokes more effective.

As mentioned earlier, almond oil is excellent as it is practically odorless and fairly inexpensive. Essential oils can be added to provide a pleasant smell and, when chosen correctly, add their own therapeutic benefits to the massage.

When massaging people who don't like the feel of oil on their skin, it is possible to use talc instead. This succeeds in making the skin smooth and slippery, but does tend to block the pores of the skin. Mineral oil has the same effect.

Lotions and creams can be used but they do not provide the smoothness of oil, can often contain additives, and may become sticky when working.

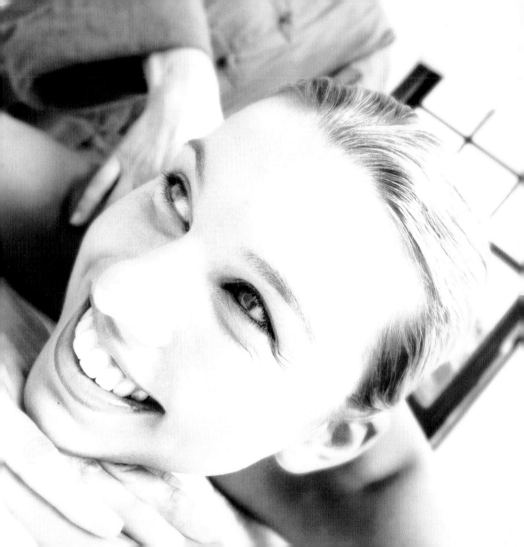

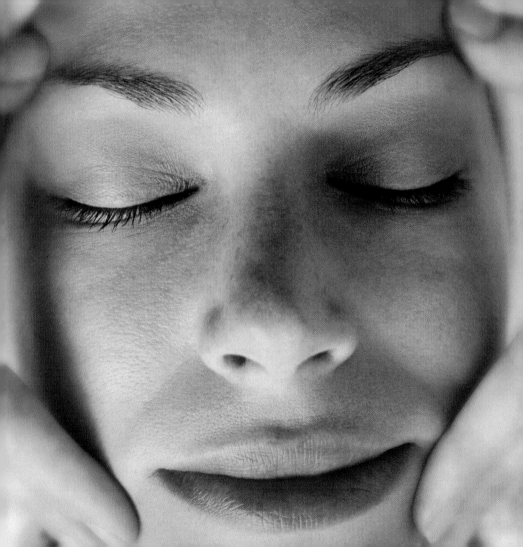

PREPARATION

CAREFUL PREPARATION OF YOUR MASSAGE ROOM IS VERY
IMPORTANT IN ORDER TO ENSURE THAT YOUR RECIPIENT GETS
THE GREATEST BENEFIT FROM YOUR MINISTRATIONS!

Choose a quiet, draft-free room with gentle lighting and make sure that light does not fall onto the recipient's face. The room needs to be really warm as oil cools the skin and people can become very cold during a massage. It is a good idea to have some soft, warm towels available so that any exposed areas of the body can be covered when they are not being worked on.

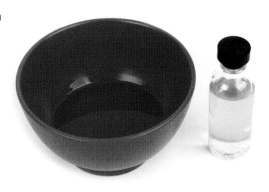

Make sure your oil is mixed, placed in a suitable container and warmed up prior to use.

Allow plenty of room for moving around the couch or padding as you will need to work on all sides.

Some people like to have gentle music playing during a massage while others prefer silence.

Before you begin your massage sequence you need to apply the oil. This should be poured a little at a time onto your hands, before being applied to the recipient. Applying directly to the recipient will give an unpleasant sensation and does not allow the oil to be checked for warmth prior to application.

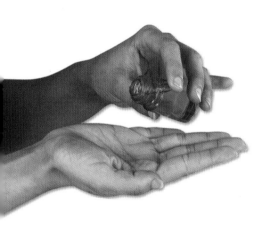

If the oil is cool you can then warm it by rubbing your hands together. Only apply oil to the area that you intend to work on first, or it will be absorbed before you can use it.

Apply the oil with both hands, covering the entire area (without leaving gaps) using a gentle stroking motion. Try not to use too much at once. It is easy to add more oil but harder to remove excess.

Bear in mind that people with more body hair need more oil, or you will pull their hair when you massage. Be careful where you put your oil bottle because while you want it easily accessible, you don't want to knock it over.

It is a golden rule of massage that, once you have made contact with the recipient's body, you should not break that contact until the end of the massage. If you need to replenish the oil or move to another area, make sure that one hand maintains contact throughout. The art of good massage is in the way you use your hands. Think of it as learning to listen with them—this will take practice.

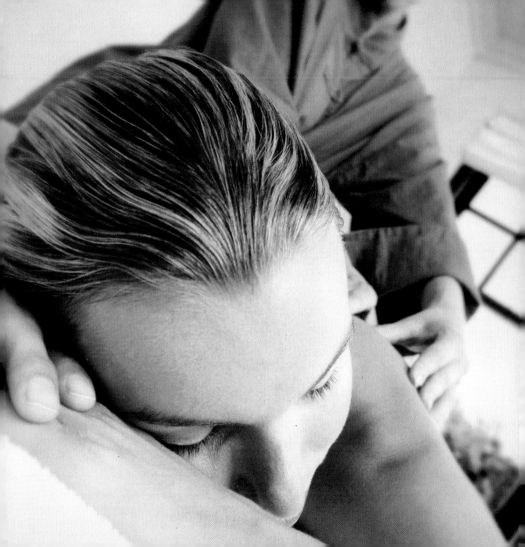

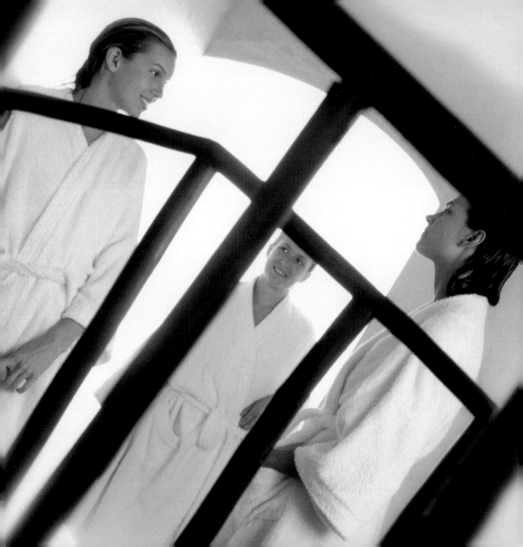

WARMING UP

IT IS IMPORTANT BEFORE GIVING A MASSAGE
THAT YOU PREPARE YOURSELF.

Firstly, wear loose and comfortable clothing, check that your fingernails are short and, if you have long hair, that it is tied back. Take off any sharp rings or jewelry and your wristwatch.

Make sure that you wash your hands thoroughly, preferably in an unscented soap, especially if you are going to use essential oils during your massage.

If you are going to have music on during the massage, make sure that it is ready. Try to prevent interruptions from the telephone and other external factors.

PREPARATION MOVES

Spend a few minutes alone before you start. Try to clear your mind of

any negativity, or thoughts about other things like the shopping list or your own stresses. It is so easy to communicate your own problems to others through touch.

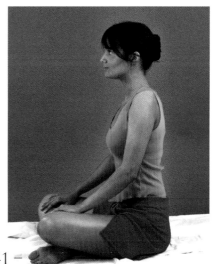

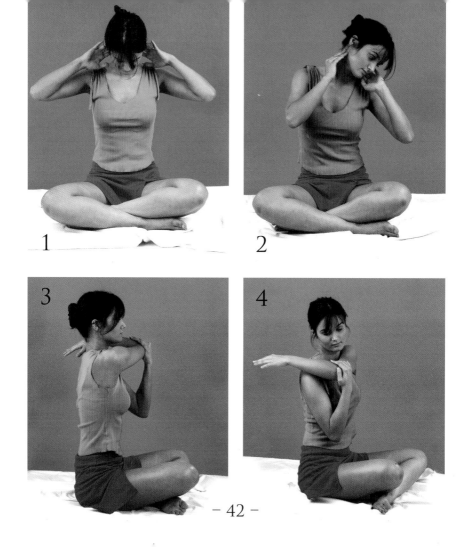

Do some slow, deep, and relaxed breathing, as during normal life we tend to breathe in a very shallow manner. Not only will it help to oxygenate your blood, it will also help you to relax.

WARM-UP EXERCISES

Try stretching your muscles by following the sequence of pictures, to ensure you are adequately warmed up. Then try to fill your mind with positive thoughts about the person you are going to massage.

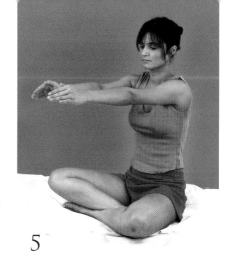

5

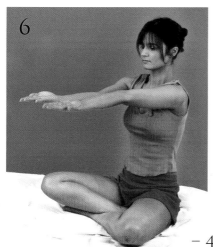

6

Your caring will help you, and them, to concentrate on the massage and make it an enjoyable and beneficial experience for both of you.

During the massage make sure your head, neck, shoulders, arms, and hands are all loose and comfortable. Your posture is important and you must remember to try to keep your back as straight as possible when you work, while also keeping your body relaxed. You should check this frequently when working.

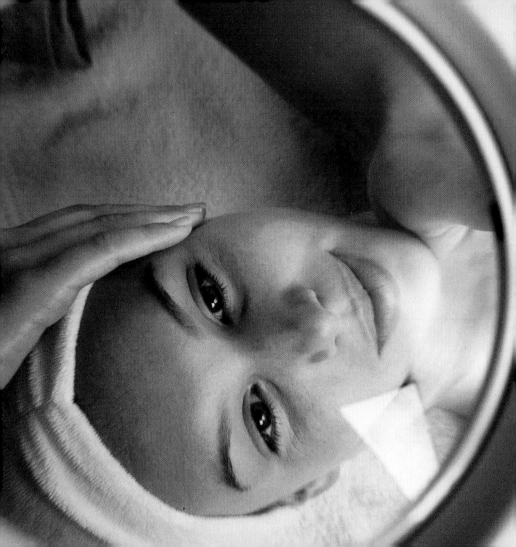

VARIOUS STROKES

IN CLASSICAL MASSAGE, MOVEMENTS ARE CLASSIFIED UNDER SIX DIFFERENT HEADINGS: EFFLEURAGE, PETRISSAGE, TAPOTEMENT, KNEADING, HACKING, AND CUPPING.

EFFLEURAGE This includes all the basic stroking movements and is done with the flat of the hand with the fingers relaxed, so they follow the contours of the body.

PETRISSAGE This is normally applied with the heel of the hand or the ball of the thumb and is applied to soft tissue that has bone underneath it.

TAPOTEMENT Refers to gentle, but rapid, vibratory movements executed with the fingers of one or both hands, usually on small muscles like those of the face.

KNEADING This is quite a deep movement that is usually applied to soft tissue where bone is not close to the surface. As the name implies, it is rather like kneading bread and is a combination of squeezing and pressing.

HACKING This movement is done using the edge of the hand with the fingers held apart. It is a bit like a chopping movement so it is important that it is always done with hands relaxed and not directly over bone.

CUPPING The hands are hollowed for this movement so that they drop onto the skin, creating a vacuum. Then, when the hands are raised, they cause suction and increase the blood flow to the skin. If executed properly, it should sound like a trotting horse.

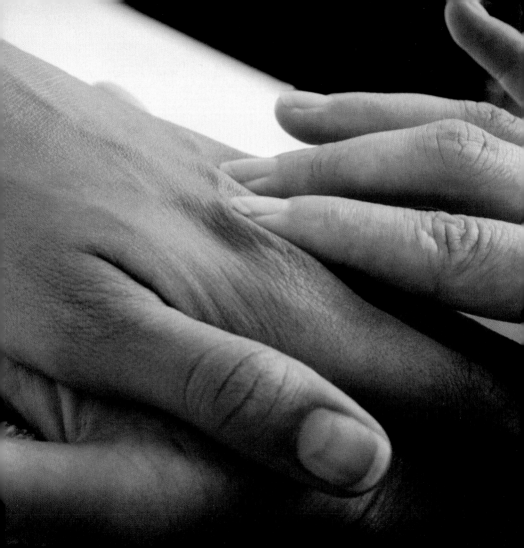

EFFLEURAGE

THESE ARE GENTLE, RHYTHMIC STROKES THAT GLIDE OVER THE SKIN. FAIRLY GENERAL MOVEMENTS, THEY ARE USED ON ALL PARTS OF THE BODY.

Effleurage strokes begin and end each massage on an individual area and can be used in between other movements to ensure smoothness and continuity.

A long stroke, formed by both hands moving slowly over the body area, can be used as a broad and soothing movement. Apart from being very relaxing, it is a good way of warming and spreading oil.

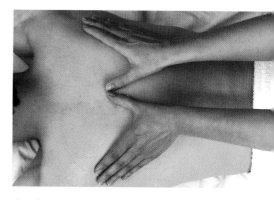

In circling, the hands move as if swimming breaststroke so that the area of the body is covered in a continuous overlapping spiral of circles. Again the hands should be relaxed so that the whole surface is in contact with the recipient.

Feathering is a very gentle movement using the fingertips in a light, brushing action. The hands are used alternately, with the touch becoming lighter and lighter. This is usually used to conclude an area or a complete massage.

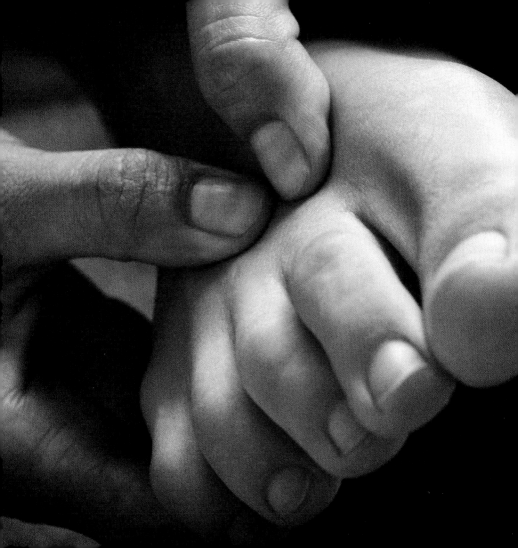

PETRISSAGE

THESE MOVEMENTS WORK ON DEEPER TISSUES AND HELP
TO RELEASE TENSION.

Thumb rolling is done by pressing the ball of the thumb into the body using small circles or short, deep strokes, and then repeating the same motion with the other thumb following behind. The leading thumb should be lifted when the other thumb is at work. By pushing along a little further each time, quite a broad area is eventually covered.

Heel-of-hand pressure is really an enlarged version of thumb rolling, with the heels of the hands used to push gently, but firmly, into the body, with one heel brought down just behind the other.

Fingertip pressure can be effective by making tiny circling movements between joints. It is important to move the underlying tissue rather than just sliding over the skin.

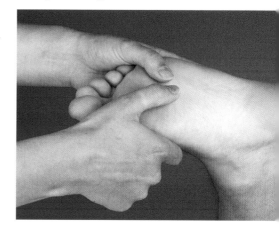

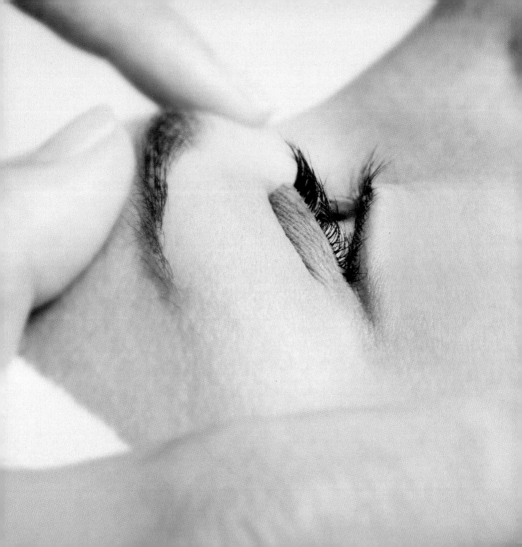

TAPOTEMENT

FAIRLY RAPID USE OF THE FINGERS ON THE SMALL MUSCLES WILL HELP RELIEVE TENSION.

The term "tapotement" comes from the French verb "tapoter," which means "'to rap, drum or pat." These movements are generally fast and stimulating and are sometimes called "percussion movements," emphasizing their rapid, rhythmic nature.

In some contexts, hacking and cupping strokes are considered tapotement movements—both administer lively, stimulating strokes that help to tone and relax the skin and muscles.

Fundamentally, the fingertips are held on a small area of flesh and vibrated from side to side, making sure that the muscle is moved. The skin and muscles are stimulated through the response of the nerves underlying the skin.

Tapotement can be light or heavy, the difference being determined by the force of the movements. To loosen tension of the face, only the superficial tissue needs to be affected.

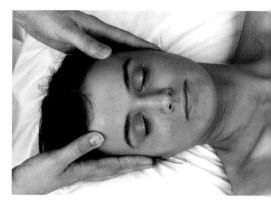

Cupping and hacking strokes are generally more forceful and result in a different type of massage.

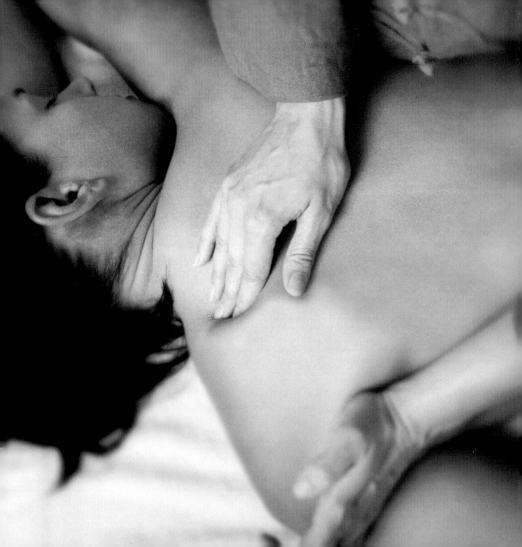

KNEADING

FOR KNEADING, USE THE WHOLE OF YOUR HANDS,
ALTERNATELY GRASPING AND SQUEEZING AREAS OF FLESH.
AS ONE HAND RELEASES ITS HOLD, THE OTHER STARTS TO
GATHER ANOTHER HANDFUL OF FLESH.

The hands should not be removed from the body between strokes but should rock smoothly back and forth, just like making bread! This is quite a broad, circular motion.

Pulling is a firm, lifting stroke used on the sides of the body, arms and legs. As you pull one hand over the body toward you, you push the other hand away from you. Continue to alternate the pull–push action while working slowly up toward the recipient's head.

Wringing is a very similar movement and is rather like a "Chinese burn" without the burn. The tissue you are working on is squeezed between the

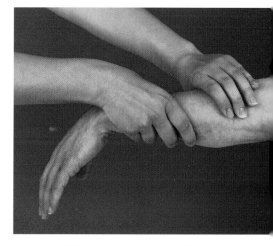

hands as if it were a wet towel. The hand should be allowed to slide a little so that there is no discomfort.

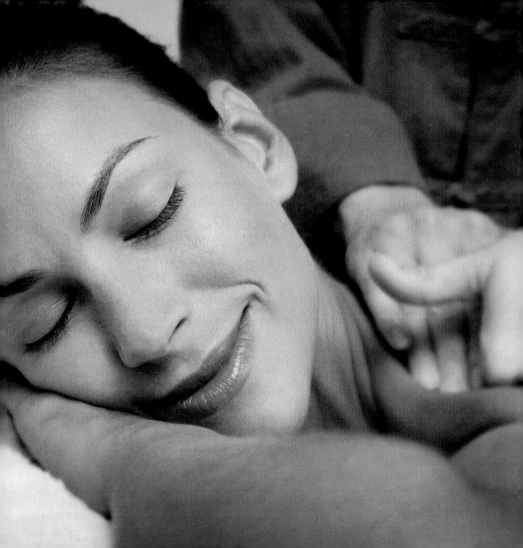

HACKING

FOR THE HACKING MOVEMENT, RELAX YOUR HANDS
BUT KEEP YOUR FINGERS APART.

With your palms facing each other, strike down toward the area of the body with the little finger of one hand.

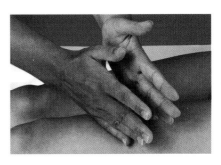

Your fingers should briefly close together before one hand bounces up as the other falls in a rapid alternating movement. It is a good idea to practice this on a cushion before trying it on bodies!

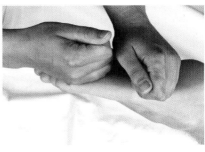

Pummeling is a similar movement but done with the hands held in loose fists and alternately dropped and bounced on and off the body. Again it should be quite rapid and rhythmic. Both these movements should be done from the wrist rather than the arm.

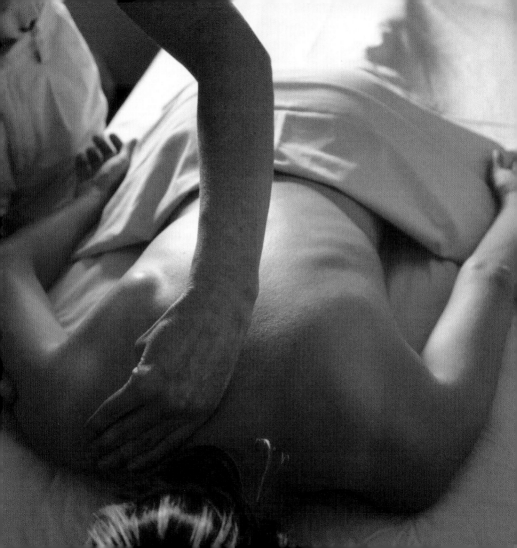

CUPPING

CUPPING IS QUITE A SIMPLE TECHNIQUE AND IS SIMILAR
TO HACKING AND PUMMELING.

Cup your hands, arching them at the
knuckles with the fingers kept
straight. Repeat the same actions
used for hacking and pummeling.

When the hand is brought down on
the body, air is expelled and creates
a vacuum. When the hand is quickly
removed this vacuum sucks blood
toward the surface of the skin.
Apart from the back, this is best used
on the more fleshy areas of the body.

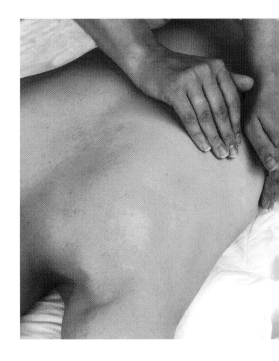

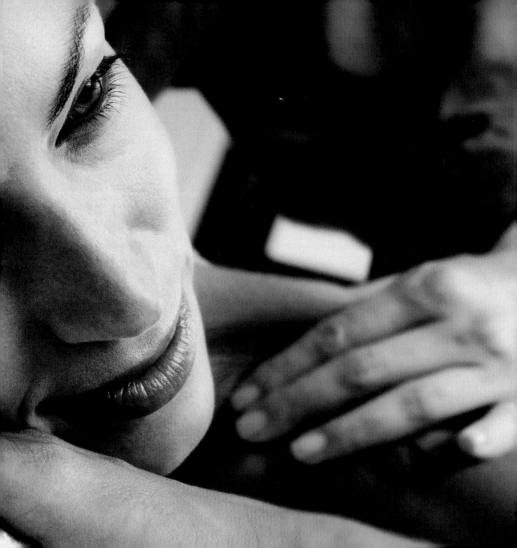

MASSAGE AREAS

THE ENTIRE BODY CAN BE CONSIDERED AS A POTENTIAL
MASSAGE AREA BUT YOU WILL FIND IT MUCH EASIER TO
CONCENTRATE ON INDIVIDUAL SECTIONS.

It really doesn't matter how many or
how few of the movements you want
to include, or how much of the body
you cover.

You can start wherever you like and
just touch individual areas if that is
more appropriate. It is usual to repeat
each movement at least three times.

Whichever area you decide to
massage, you should start and
finish with the same movement.

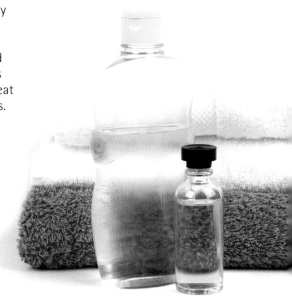

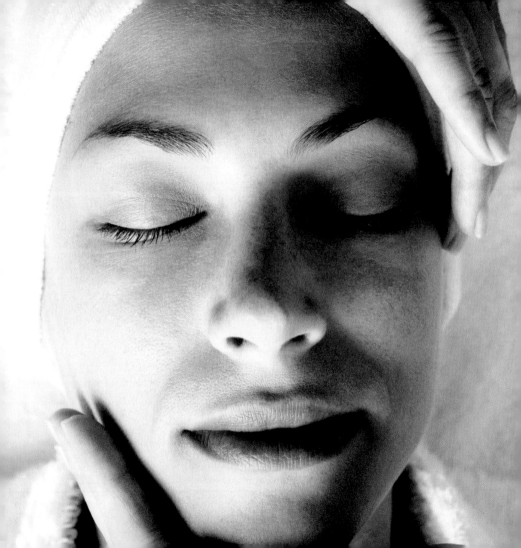

HEAD

SHAMPOOING, RUBBING THE SCALP, AND PULLING HAIR
ARE ALL EXCELLENT TECHNIQUES FOR HEAD MASSAGE.

SHAMPOOING

Turn the head to one side and support with one hand.

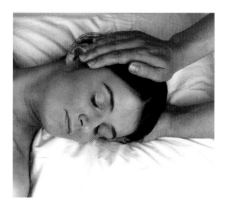

With the other hand, use the tips of the fingers to rub small circles into the scalp in one place. Do not allow your fingers to slide over the skin.

Lift the hand, move to another area and repeat until one side of the scalp has been covered.

Then, turn the head to the other side and repeat.

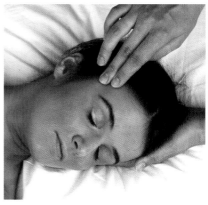

RUBBING THE SCALP

Turn the head to one side and support with one hand. Use the flat of the other hand to rub large areas of the scalp.

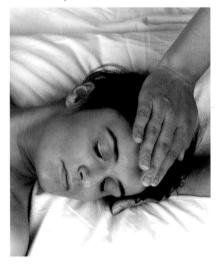

Lift the hand, move to another area and repeat until one side of the scalp has been covered. Then, turn the head to the other side and repeat.

PULLING HAIR

Taking a large bunch of hair in each hand, gently pull from the roots and release.

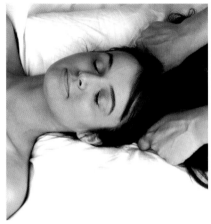

Continue working all over the head until all the hair has been pulled.

Be careful to hold plenty of hair each time and you will find that, rather than being uncomfortable, this is a very pleasant, relaxing movement.

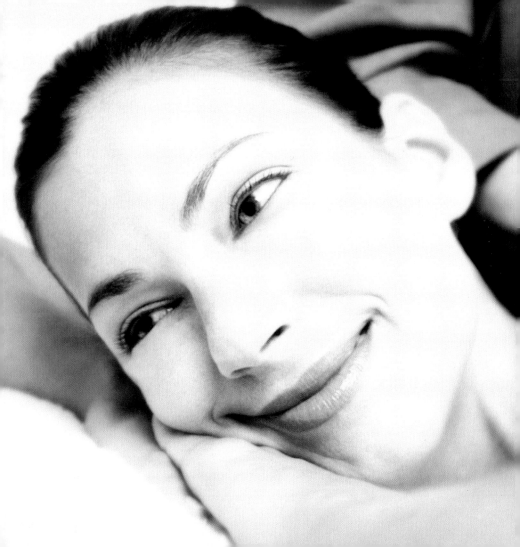

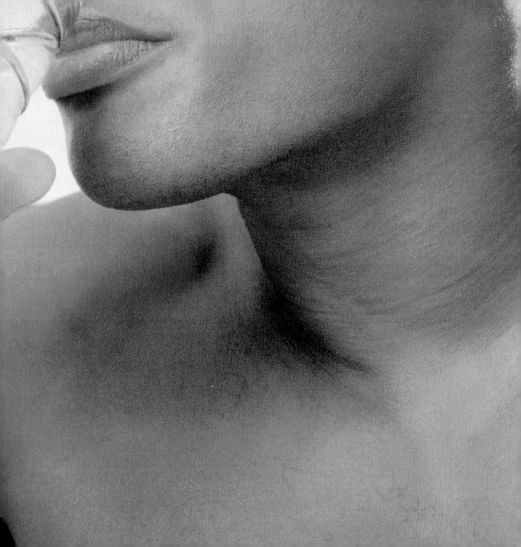

NECK

WHEN WORKING ON THE NECK, TRY TO ENSURE THAT THE RECIPIENT IS AS RELAXED AS POSSIBLE AND DO NOT ATTEMPT ANY MOVEMENTS THAT CAUSE STRAIN OF ANY SORT.

STRETCHING THE NECK
Place both hands under the neck so that your little fingers come to rest at the base of the skull while your hands provide support.

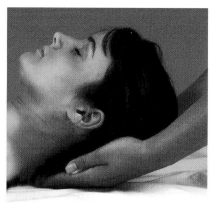

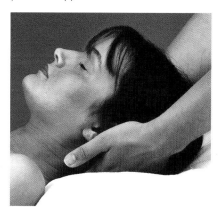

Lift the neck slightly from the work surface and pull toward you so that you stretch the neck backwards and straight. Gently release and lower the head.

LIFTING THE NECK

Place both hands under the neck so that your little fingers come to rest at the base of the skull while your hands support the neck.

Gently and slowly, lift the head and bring the chin toward the chest. Hold the position briefly before gently lowering the head again.

Then, move your hands down the neck so that they are now under the hollow.

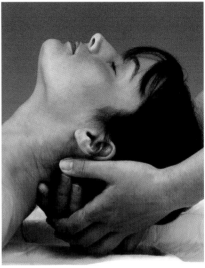

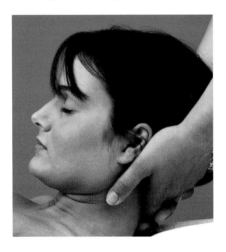

Lift the neck so that the head drops backward. Then, slide your hands back to the base of the skull, pull gently and lower the head.

STRETCHING THE NECK SIDEWAYS

With one hand under the neck, hold the base of the skull securely.

Lift the head slightly and slowly move it toward one shoulder while pushing gently on the opposite shoulder with your other hand.

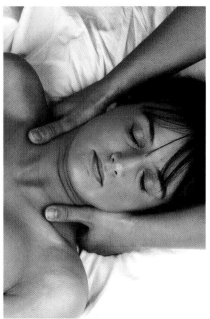

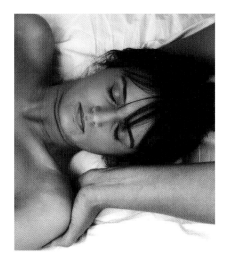

Release the pressure on the shoulder and gently return the head to the center. Change hands and repeat on the other side.

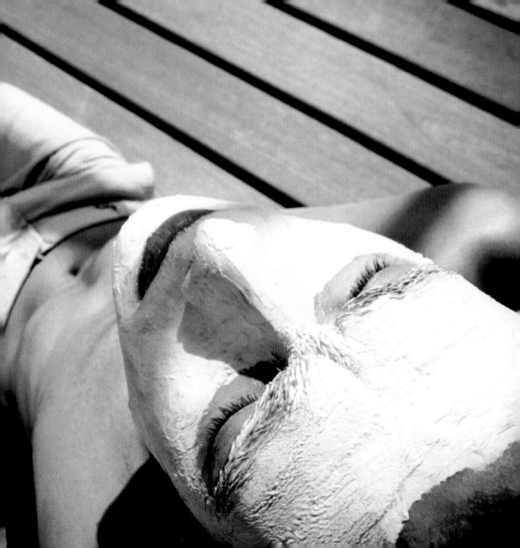

FACE

PEOPLE WILL REALLY ENJOY A FACE MASSAGE
AS IT FEELS LIKE A GREAT LUXURY.

FOREHEAD

Cupping the scalp in both hands, place your thumbs at the center of the forehead, just below the hairline.

Move your thumbs slowly apart to each side of the forehead. Lift the thumbs and return to the center.

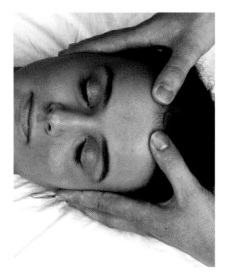

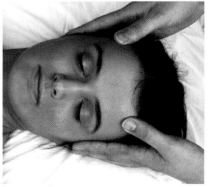

Move the thumbs down and repeat so that the forehead is massaged in "strips" until the whole surface has been covered.

EYEBROWS

Cupping the scalp in both hands, place your thumbs in the center of the head at the beginning of the eyebrows.

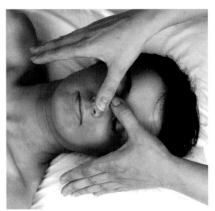

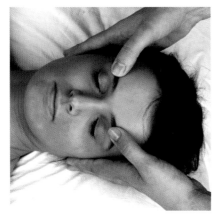

Move your thumbs slowly apart, covering the whole eyebrow line.

NOSE

Using your thumbs alternately, stroke down from the bridge of the nose to the tip.

Then stroke one side of the nose from the bridge to the tip and then the other side. Repeat three times.

CHEEKS

Place one hand on each side of the face. Beginning just under the inner corners of the eyes, stroke your thumbs across the face and down toward the ears. Bring your thumbs back and repeat this, moving down in small sections at a time.

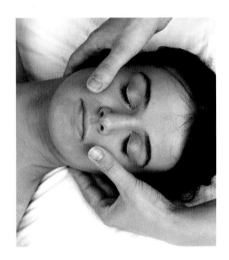

Gradually moving your hands apart, work along the whole chin and along the lower jaw as far as the ears.

Lastly, slide your hands smoothly down the face, across the cheeks, and under the ears to the back of the neck. Pull your hands up the neck and under the back of the head toward you. Let your hands slide over the head and the hair.

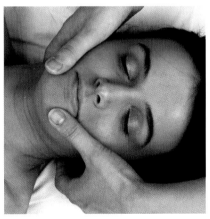

Continue the movement below the nose over the top lip, below the mouth under the bottom lip, and continue down to the chin until the whole face has been covered.

CHIN

Hold the point of the chin between your thumbs and index fingers and gently squeeze and release.

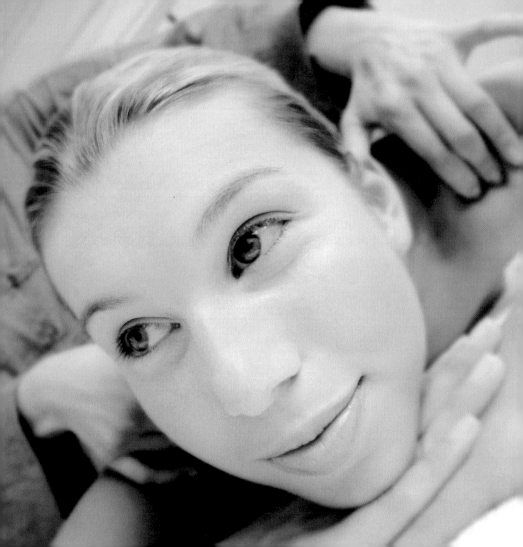

SHOULDERS

A SHOULDER MASSAGE IS GREAT FOR RELIEVING TENSION.

Position yourself at the recipient's head. Place your hands on the upper chest just below the collarbone with your fingers pointing toward each other. Slowly draw your hands apart with the heels of your hands pointing toward the shoulders.

Keeping your hands relaxed, stroke over and right around the shoulder joint until you come to the neck. Slide your hands up the neck before gently moving them back to the center of the chest without losing contact.

Turn your recipent over and, working from the side, hold one arm of the recipient. With your other hand, hold the shoulder joint and lift it slightly. Then, using both your hands, rotate the joint in slow circles round and round, moving as far as possible down, up and toward the neck in a clockwise direction. Then, repeat the movement in the opposite direction.

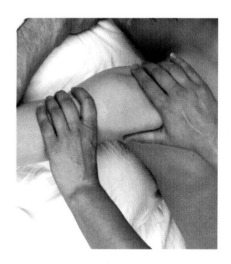

ARMS

FOR ARM MASSAGE YOU WILL NEED TO PRODUCE
A "WRINGING" MOTION.

Working from the side, let your hands rest on the recipient's wrist with your fingers pointing upward. Whichever of your hands is nearest the head should lead.

With your hands at the wrist, lift and pull the tissues with the fingers of the leading hand while pushing away with the thumb of the other.

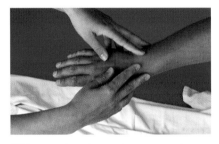

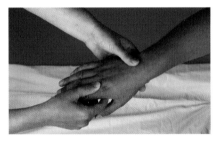

Slide your hands up the arm to the top. Let your leading hand stroke over the shoulder joint while the other hand slides down just under the armpit. Then, allowing your hands to hold as much of the arm as possible, slide your hands back down to the wrist.

Release and reverse so that the thumb of the leading hand pushes against the fingers of the other. This produces the "wringing" motion. Gradually work all the way up the arm to the armpit in a steady rhythm. On arrival at the top, slide both hands back to the wrist and repeat.

Lift the arm so that it bends at the elbow and allow it to rest against you. With your hands at the wrist use alternate thumbs to push along, sideways and toward the elbow, gradually moving along the arm.

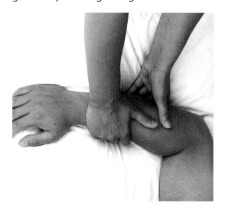

When you reach the elbow, slide the hands back to the wrist. Gently squeeze your hand together around the arm and, in a continuous movement, push toward the elbow. Slide your hands back to the wrist and repeat.

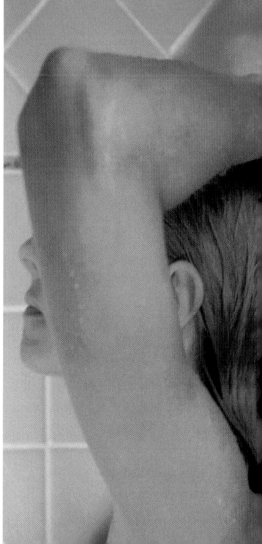

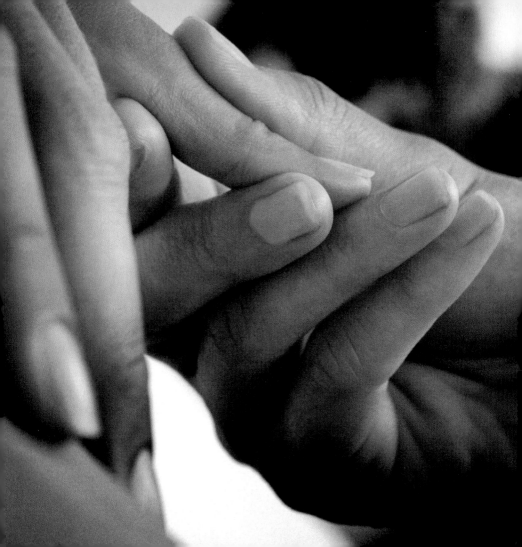

HANDS

Use your thumbs alternately, working in small circles over the back of the wrist area while holding the wrist between your thumbs and fingers.

Using your thumbs alternately, start at the base of the fingers, pushing down and out to stroke and stretch the palm in a steady rhythm.

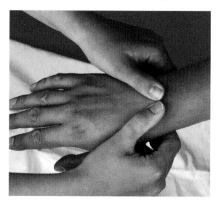

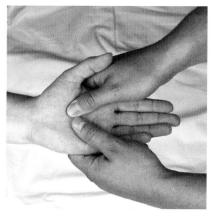

Then turn the recipient's hand gently and repeat on the front of the wrist and continue the movement into the palm of the hand.

Now, turn the hand over and repeat this on the back of the hand between the bones and tendons.

Take the recipient's thumb, and each finger in turn, between your fingers and thumb.

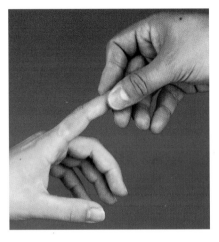

Using your thumb, make small circles along the length of each digit from the base to the tip while gently pulling. When you arrive at the end of the digit, slide back to the base and along to the tip in a continuous movement.

Hold the recipient's wrist in one hand and interlink the fingers of your other hand with theirs. Slowly rotate their hand in the largest clockwise circles you can comfortably achieve a few times, and then reverse.

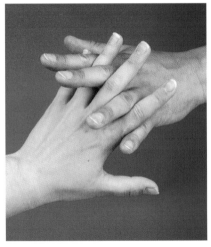

If you have decided to massage a whole hand you should repeat the first movement at the end.

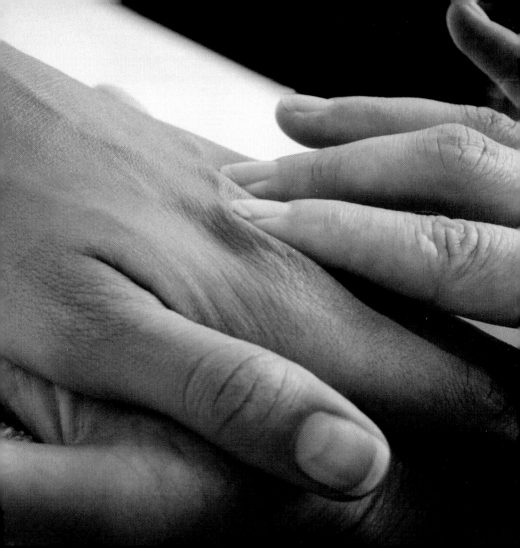

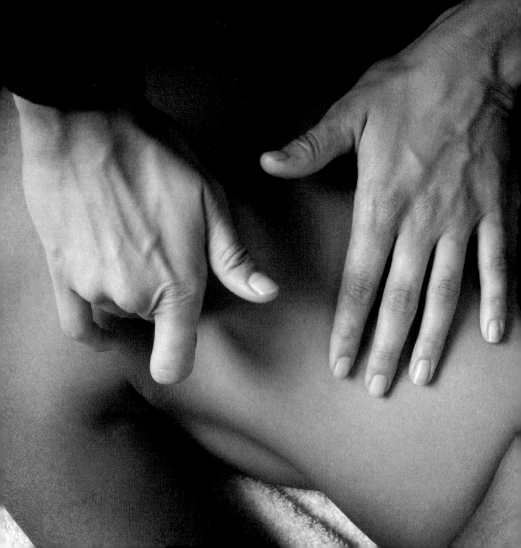

BACK

THE BACK CAN HOLD A LOT OF TENSION SO
WILL BENEFIT FROM A SLOW, FIRM MASSAGE.

Place your hands on either side of
the top of the back with your
thumbs pointing toward each other.

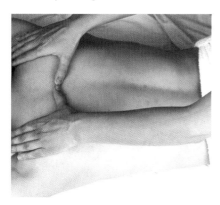

Using a firm pressure, glide down the
entire length of the back, gradually
bringing your fingers together.

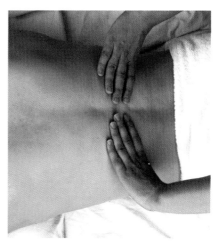

Separate your hands when you near
the lower end of the spine, leading
them over and down the sides of
the hips.

Then, slowly push the hands along the side of the torso in the direction of the shoulders.

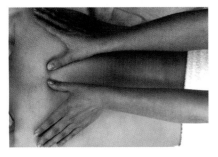

Just before reaching the armpits, glide your hands back onto the top of the back and pivot them so that the fingers point toward each other.

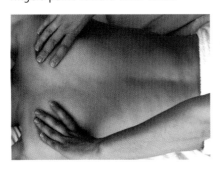

This movement should begin and end any back massage and can always be repeated between other movements.

From the side, place one hand at one side of the base of the spine so that the ball of your thumb lies in the groove beside it. Place your other hand on top. Work up the back from the base to the head, making circles with your hands.

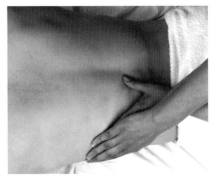

The idea is to push the muscle away from the spine upward and outward to the side. Keep your pressure moderate and steady throughout.

When you arrive at the top of the spine, slide your hands back to the base and repeat. Then, repeat the movement on the other side of the spine.

Still from the side, place one hand at the side of the back below the shoulder blade and place your other hand on top. Slide your hands out to the side, under, and around the shoulder joint and under the large muscle at the base of the neck. Lift and pull the muscle with your hands toward the back, allowing your hands to slide slowly over it and back to the middle. Then, continue the movement to the other side so that you are effectively making a figure of eight around the recipient's shoulders.

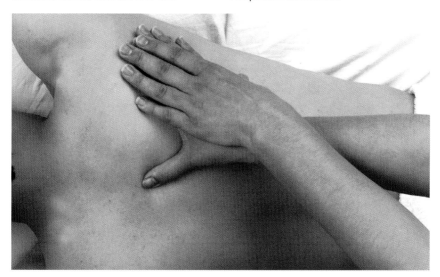

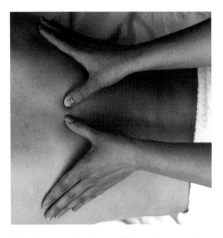

opposite you. With each stroke of your hands, grasp the loose flesh between your fingers and thumbs and let it slowly slip between them while feeding it into the other hand.

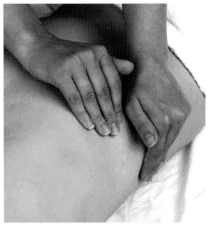

Starting at the base of the spine, make short, deep circles with your thumbs pointing upward on either side of the spine. Stop and press briefly in between each of the bones of the spinal column as you work your way up to the top then slide your hands back down to the base.

From the side, knead the back from the waist to the shoulders and back again. Reach across to the side

Your hands should alternate, beginning a new stroke with one hand slightly before finishing a stroke with the other. This becomes a rhythmic motion in which the hands are always moving.

Work up the outside of the back and down the middle a few times before moving to do the same on the other side.

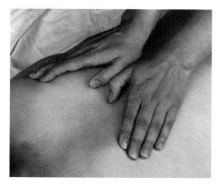

Again from the side, run your hands in horizontal strips across the back. Reach over the back with one hand, keeping the other hand on the side nearest you. As you push with one hand, you pull with the other so that your hands pass each other over the spine and your hands change places. Repeat this movement as you move down to the base of the back and then back up again.

Done slowly this is a very relaxing movement for the recipient or, if done rapidly, it can produce a lot of friction and warming.

From the side, using two fingers of one hand, trace down the length of the spine, from neck to waist. When your hand gets near the base, start the movement again with the other hand and repeat. Continue this, using alternate hands with your pressure becoming lighter and lighter with each stroke. If your recipient has not fallen asleep yet, they will now!

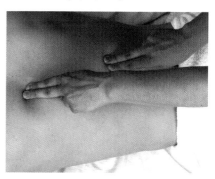

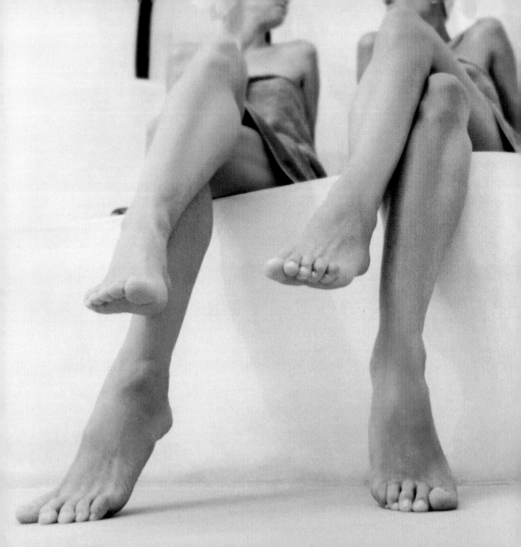

LEGS

LEG MASSAGE IS SIMILAR TO ARM MASSAGE AND IS
DEFINITELY ONE TECHNIQUE YOU SHOULD MASTER.

Place yourself at the feet and slightly to one side of your recipient and move their feet roughly a foot (thirty centimeters) apart. Put whichever of your hands is nearest their outer thigh just above the ankle, with your fingertips pointing toward the inside of the leg. Place your other hand just below, with the fingers pointing to the outside of the leg.

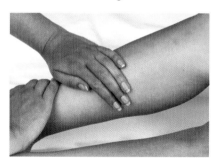

Pressing firmly, move both hands together up the leg, releasing the pressure slightly as you move over the knee.

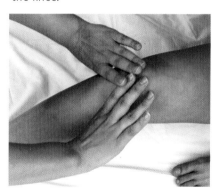

Separate your hands, allowing your leading hand to stroke round the top of the thigh, while the other moves down below the groin.

Then bring the hands back down the sides of the legs to the ankle, pulling gently as you go. As your hands near the ankle, return them to the starting position.

From the side, place both hands side by side across the base of the calf muscle with your fingers pointing away from you. Keep as much of your hands in contact as possible.

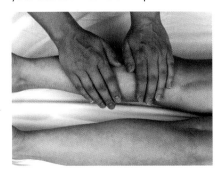

Move your left hand away from you and down, maintaining full contact with the leg, until the fingertips touch the work surface. At the same time move your right hand toward

you and down, until the heel of the hand also reaches the work surface.

Next, while pushing the hands toward each other to put pressure on the leg, move both hands in the reverse direction.

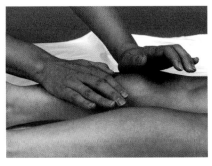

Keep alternating like this, gradually working to the top of the leg. When you reach the top, return your hands in the same way as you did for the previous movement.

Place your palms against either side of the foreleg right at the ankle. Have as much of your hands in contact as possible. Place your thumbs at the front of the leg with your fingers pointing toward the back.

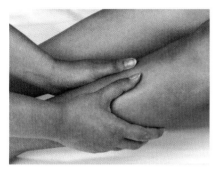

Slowly glide both hands up the leg, squeezing them together. Release the pressure over the knee and increase it again for the upper leg. When you get to the top, return to the ankle in the same way.

From the side, knead the back of the leg from the ankle to the top and then reach across to the side opposite you. With each stroke of your hands, grasp the loose flesh between your fingers and thumbs and let it slowly

slip between them while feeding it into the other hand.

As before, your hands should alternate, beginning a new stroke with one hand slightly before finishing a stroke with the other. By keeping the hands always moving you should be able to create a rhythmic motion. Work up the inside of the leg first and then down the outside.

When one leg is completed, repeat the same movements on the other leg. All these movements can be used on the front and back of the legs.

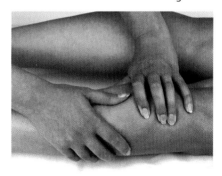

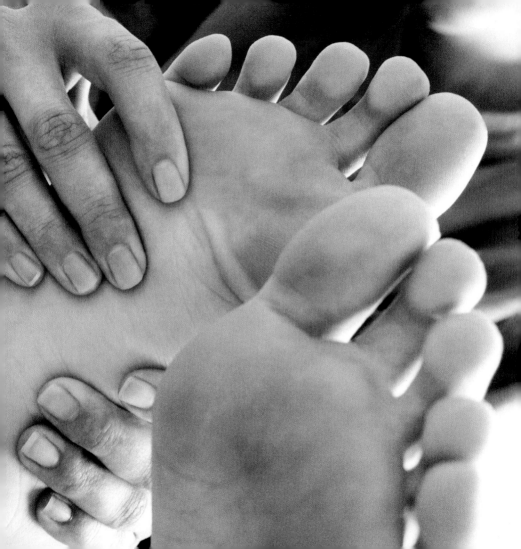

FEET

From the side, place your hands as if praying and clasp the foot between them so that your thumbs are by the big toe. One palm should rest upon the top of the foot, while the other supports the sole.

Slide your hands down along the length of the foot toward the ankle, allowing your fingers to curl as you near the work surface and then return to the beginning, doing a circular motion around the whole foot.

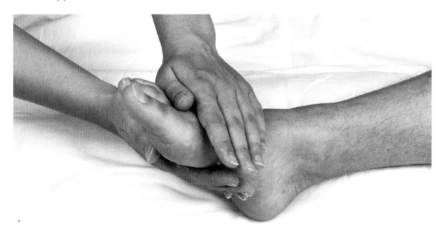

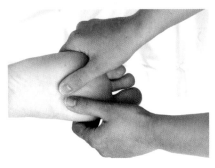

Use your thumbs in the same way to massage the top of the foot, working between the tendons and bones.

Using the tips of your fingers of both hands, circle the ankle bone on both the inside and outside at the same time.

Hold the foot in place with your fingers and, with alternating thumbs, work on the sole of the foot using small circles and pushing down toward the ankle. Continue until the whole surface has been covered.

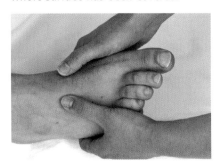

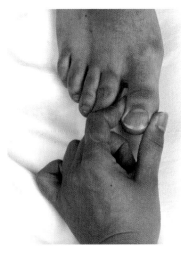

Take each of the recipient's toes in turn between your finger and thumb.

Using your thumb, make small circles from the base to the tip of each digit while gently pulling.

Hold the recipient's ankle in one hand and hold the foot with your other hand.

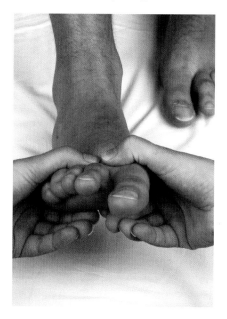

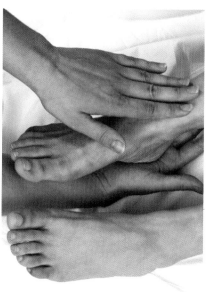

When you arrive at the end of the digit, slide back to the base and along to the tip in a continuous movement.

Slowly rotate their foot in the largest clockwise circles you can comfortably achieve a few times and then reverse.

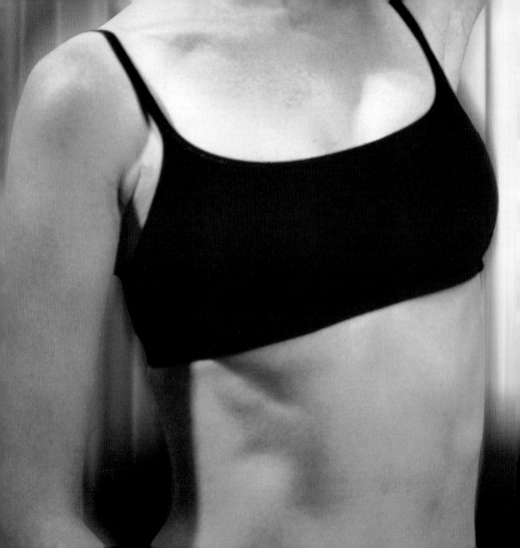

ABDOMEN

IT'S IMPORTANT TO BE GENTLE WHEN MASSAGING
THIS PART OF THE BODY.

Gently rest your hands side by side on the recipient's belly.

Then, lift and pull both hands together to return them to the middle.

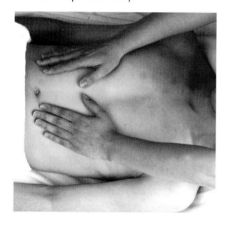

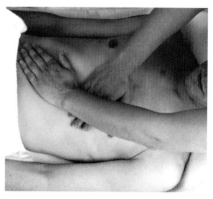

Slide your hands together down the front toward the pelvis, then up to just below the rib cage where they should separate, one going to each side and dropping beside the waist.

From the center, move both hands clockwise over the belly, letting them flow over the contours. One hand can complete whole circles, but the other will have to break contact each time the hands cross.

Continue to move in a clockwise direction, making very small circular movements all round the edges of the belly.

As the recipient inhales and the chest rises, slide your hands up the center of the torso to the base of the ribcage.

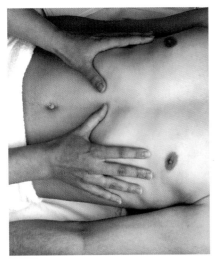

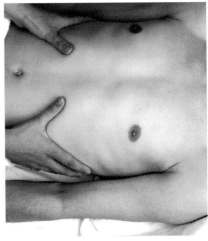

Facing the head, rest your hands on the belly with your fingers pointing up the body.

As the recipient exhales and the chest falls, move your hands across to the sides before bringing them back to the center.

Leaning across from the side, run your hands in horizontal strips across the abdomen.

As you push with one hand, you pull with the other so that your hands pass each other over the belly and change places.

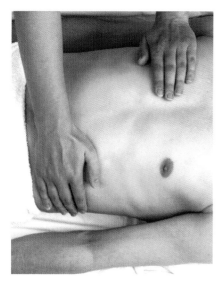

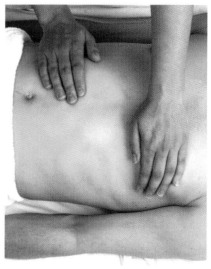

Reach over with one hand, keeping the other hand on the side nearest to you.

You should then repeat this movement several times.

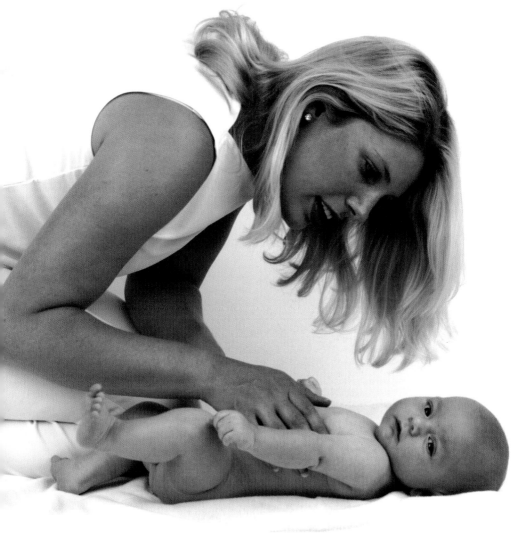

BABY MASSAGE

BABY MASSAGE CAN STRENGTHEN THE BOND
BETWEEN INFANT AND ADULT.

All of us enjoy touch, as it is not only a vital form of communication, but also an important factor in the binding process of families and couples all over the animal kingdom.

The various different massage movements described in this book are suitable for babies. It is really just a matter of using the same, or similar, movements but reducing everything in size and intensity to fit the smaller package! It is, however, worth considering a few additional guidelines.

Keep the room in which a baby is massaged very warm as they tend to lose heat more quickly than adults and are not able to regulate their own temperature so efficiently.

Babies wriggle and fidget, so it may well be worth acquiring the assistance of the favorite teddy or cuddly toy.

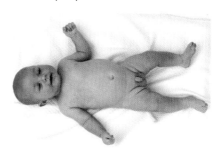

WARNING:
THE OILS CONTAINED IN THIS PACK ARE NOT SUITABLE FOR USE ON BABIES AND CHILDREN.

Don't feel that you have to be too gentle. Babies are very resilient creatures; they have to be to grow into adults. Too gentle a touch can be ticklish but obviously you don't want to use so much pressure that it becomes painful. So, aim at light to medium pressure for the optimum response.

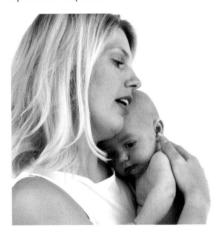

Babies can be massaged soon after birth, but adjust your movements accordingly. However, massage of the abdomen should only be conducted once the belly button has healed.

On a very small baby it may well prove easier to massage them between your legs, with the head either pointing toward, or away from you.

Instead of using your whole hand, you could just use two or three fingers, or your thumb. You need to scale everything down to fit the size you are working on.

Children are often much more open to massage than adults as they haven't learnt the inhibitions adults accumulate. If you start them early and they enjoy the process they may well repay you in later life!

When massaging babies it is best to stick to a good quality carrier oil. Alternatively you could use a proprietary baby oil, which can be easily bought from a local store or pharmacy.

Aim to spend about ten minutes on the massage routine. Half an hour after a meal, or after a bath are good times to begin as your baby should already be in a relatively calm state.

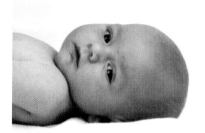

FACE

Using a small amount of oil, position your baby on his back and place your hands side by side on his forehead. Gently stroke outward, then repeat, stroking over the eyebrows and the temples back round to under the eyes.

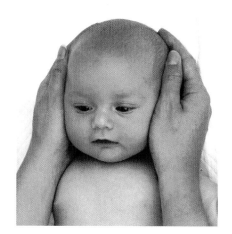

Move your hands down the nose and over the cheeks to the chin. Carefully repeat these movements as appropriate.

Gently stroke your baby's hand then take each finger in turn and rotate it.

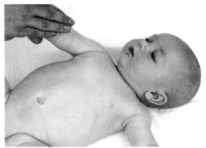

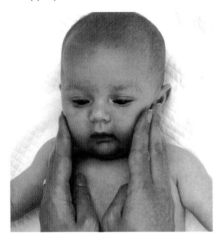

Repeat the same movements for the legs. At the end of the massaging of each limb, slightly bend and stretch the arm or leg.

ARMS AND LEGS

Take each arm in turn and slowly stroke downward, hand over hand, from the shoulder down to the hand. As you move downward, gently use a squeezing or pulling motion.

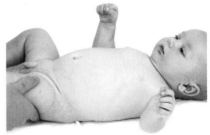

ABDOMEN AND SHOULDERS

With your open palm, massage the stomach in a clockwise direction. Follow each circular movement with the second hand, ensuring that neither stroke exerts too much downward pressure. Increase the sweeping movement of each stroke to incorporate the chest and shoulders, bringing your hands round and down the arms, and down the side of the body. A good way to finish the movement is to alternate with each hand to stroke down from the shoulders over the chest.

BACK

With your baby lying on his stomach, use gentle movements over the backs of the legs and the buttocks. Some babies may respond to soft patting or pinching. Develop the movement into a broader stroke to cover the back and the shoulders. Sweep back down along the sides and repeat. At the base of the spine, and up either side, use a slow-moving clockwise massage. With alternate hands, finish by stroking from the head down over the back to the feet.

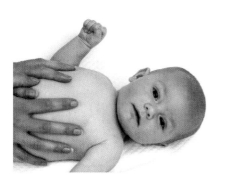

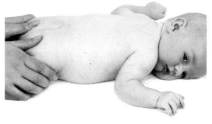

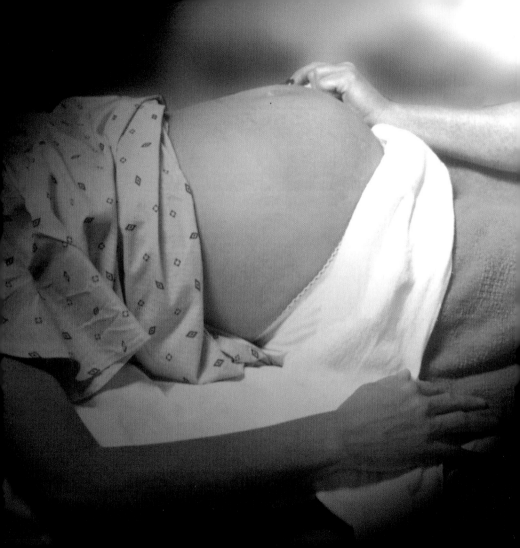

STRETCH MARKS

IT IS WELL WORTH INDULGING IN SOME MASSAGE
DURING THE LAST FOUR MONTHS OF PREGNANCY.

During the later stages of pregnancy, massage will help avoid the problem of stretch marks. The areas most affected are the tummy, thighs, buttocks, and breasts.

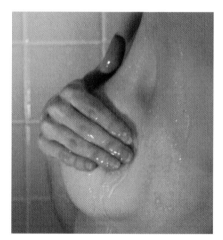

The abdominal massage is quite suitable to use up until the final stages of pregnancy. Use the broader, stroking movements with the full hand on the thighs, buttocks and breasts.

Add to your basic massage oil about ten per cent of cold-pressed wheatgerm oil and some lavender oil. If you can afford it, neroli or orange blossom oil are both marvelous, and if these aren't available, mandarin or petitgrain are both really helpful.

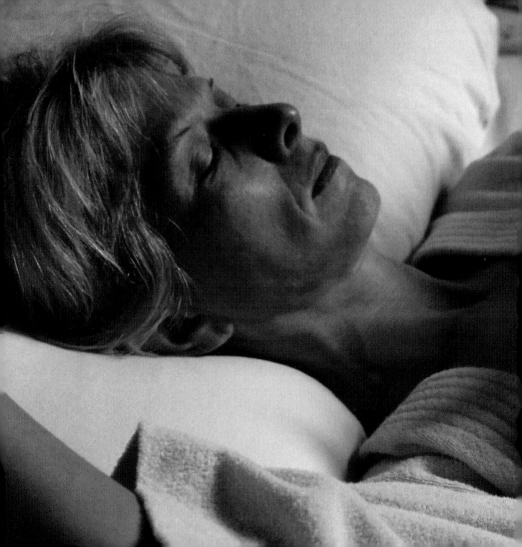

INSOMNIA

IF YOUR PARTNER HAS TROUBLE SLEEPING, IT IS LIKELY TO
AFFECT YOU AS WELL. THE ADDITION OF ESSENTIAL OILS
TO A MASSAGE MAY OFFER A SOLUTION.

Facial and back massages are very
effective ways of getting people to
relax and the addition of essential
oils can take this one step further.

Lavender, neroli, and chamomile are
great favorites and have the
additional benefit of calming the
mind and emotions, helping to
alleviate some anxiety.

Other oils to consider include
marjoram, sandalwood, or ylang
ylang, although the latter needs to
be used sparingly.

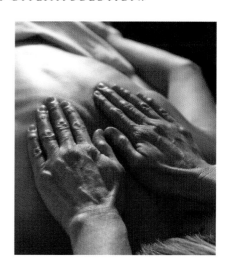

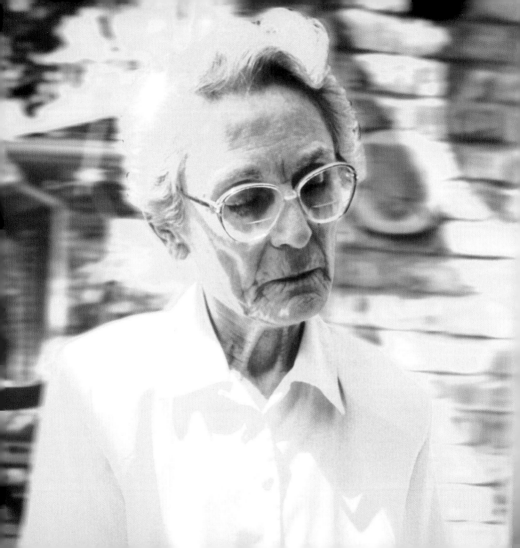

ELDERLY/RECUPERATIVE MASSAGE

IF YOU'RE SUFFERING FROM POOR CIRCULATION, A HANGOVER, OR JETLAG, A MASSAGE WITH OIL CAN WORK WONDERS.

Leg massage can be tremendously beneficial for circulation as it helps to improve the removal of the body's natural waste products and the build-up of fluid.

Try adding some rosemary and frankincense oils, especially in the case of the elderly recipient.

Cypress can be effective if fluid is the problem and cedarwood is very good for itchiness.

Bear in mind though that you should never massage over varicose veins and elderly recipients may need to consult a doctor first.

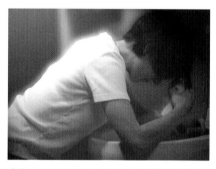

A hangover can be helped with a facial or a back massage, and the addition of neroli or petitgrain oils will speed up your recovery. Trusty lavender may come to the rescue again and marjoram can help that dreadful headache. Pay particular attention to the forehead and temples when doing the massage.

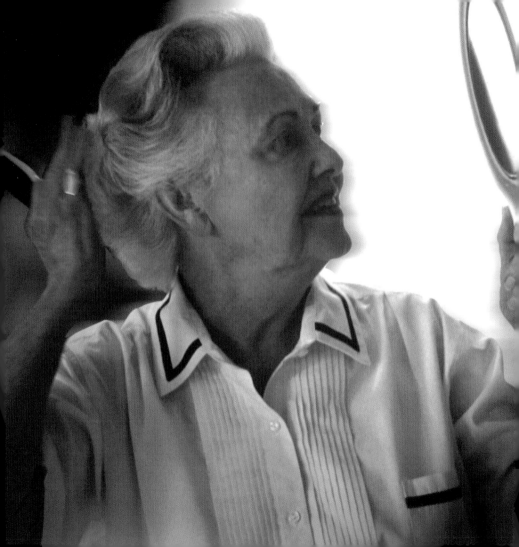

WRINKLES

KEEP YOUR YOUNG LOOKS WITH A DASH OF JOJOBA OR PEACH KERNEL OIL.

A facial massage is a good way to help alleviate wrinkles but add some jojoba to your massage oil, or splash out on some peach kernel oil as your base. You will wonder why you ever spent so much money on cosmetics that claim to help!

The very nature of massage stimulates the nerve endings that will help to tone and tighten the skin. The addition of evening primrose oil is thought to help with premature aging and it will certainly help dry skin. Geranium oil will assist problems such as eczema and acne.

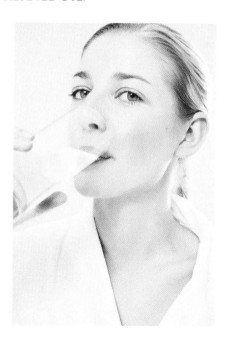

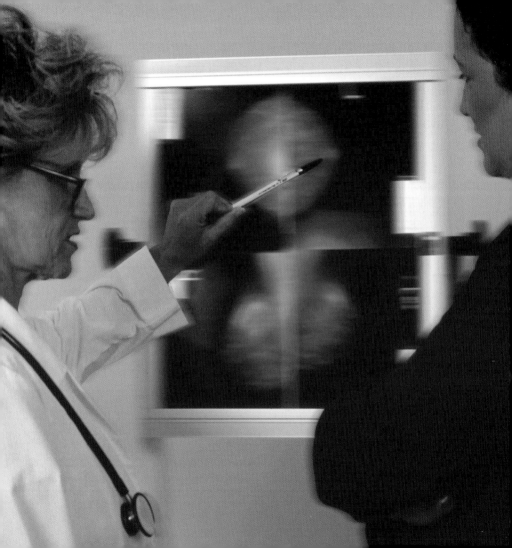

POST-SURGERY/ GENERAL INJURIES

DON'T FORGET THAT MASSAGE, WHEN EXECUTED WELL, PROVIDES A FORM OF PASSIVE EXERCISE.

Massage can be beneficial to those who have suffered an injury, or have had surgery, and can help them to recover more quickly. Before using any form of massage to aid recuperation, always consult your doctor.

One of the major problems following a variety of chest operations or injuries is a build-up of fluid in the arms. The arm massage movements can be really beneficial in helping to clear this. You can add some cypress, lavender, or juniper oil to your base oil in small amounts. All will help get your body back into working order.

Add lavender to your massage oil, as it is wonderful for so many conditions. Add some black pepper if there is any nerve damage, or cypress if there is a build-up of fluid in the tissues.

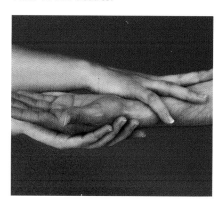

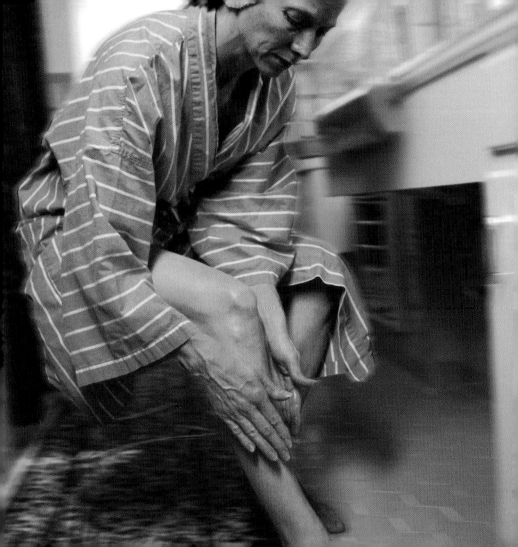

SELF-MASSAGE

SELF-MASSAGE CAN BE INCREDIBLY EFFECTIVE
AND IS FREE AS WELL!

If you hit your head, are stiff, in pain, or have hurt some part of your body, you rub it. This rubbing is a simple form of self-massage.

No one knows your body as well as you and in some ways you are therefore the best person to perform the massage. You know where you feel discomfort and how the pressure feels better than anyone.

The disadvantages are that it is hard to relax completely and difficult to reach some parts of the body without straining. The obstacles are, however, definitely outweighed by the rewards and it is one of the best ways of learning how to be a good masseur.

You will be able to massage whichever parts of the body you can reach by using, or adapting, the basic massage strokes in this book. You will probably find it easiest to relax if you treat each area as suggested here.

Start each area with a gentle touch and gradually apply more pressure, experimenting with different movements. Give yourself enough time to work on all areas, so that you feel relaxed and revitalized at the end.

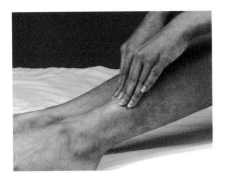

Work on the feet first, then the ankles and lower legs, over and around the knees and lastly from the knees to the hips.

HIPS AND ABDOMEN
Lie down with your knees up and massage the pelvic area from the pubic bone between the legs to the buttocks.

LEGS AND FEET
Sit on the floor with your legs in front of you and alternate between the right and left sides, starting with the right. This will help with your natural lymphatic drainage system.

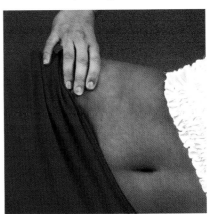

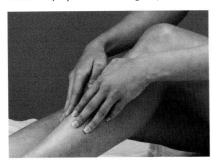

Roll over onto one side and massage the buttock surface, around the hip bone and joint with the leg. Repeat on the other side.

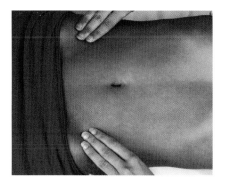

While lying down, massage the abdomen by adapting movements from pages 94–97.

CHEST
Still lying down, massage from the stomach to the collarbone.

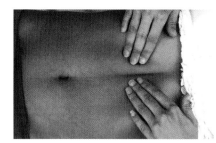

Then, pull upward from the waist along the sides of your chest. Using your fingertips, work between the ribs from the midline outward to the sides.

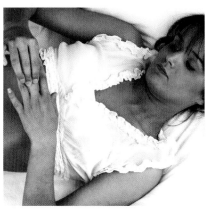

ARMS AND HANDS
Lying down, start with the right arm and massage the hand. Take time over each finger, then the wrist, forearm, and round the elbow joint. Finally, massage the upper arms to the armpits and around the shoulder joint. Repeat the movements on the left arm.

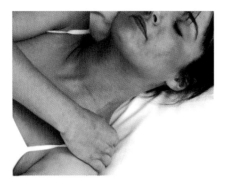

Massage the muscles across the shoulders one side at a time. You will find squeezing these very beneficial.

Then massage the sides and back of the neck and as much of the shoulder blades and upper back as you can reach without straining.

SHOULDERS AND NECK

Lying down, use your fingertips to work along the edges of the collarbone from the midline to the arms.

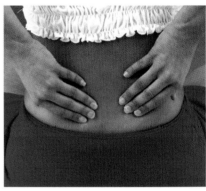

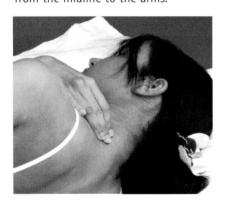

BACK

By sitting up straight, you can reach a substantial amount of this area. The lower back can be massaged using both hands while the remainder is best attempted one side at a time.

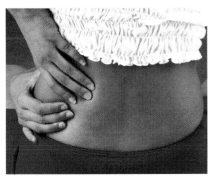

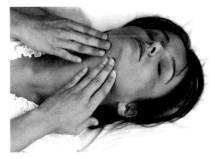

FACE AND HEAD

Lying down, start by stroking the whole face quite firmly. Begin in the center of the forehead and stroke outward to the temples.

Work all the way down the face to the chin. Massage the jaw and the ears and finish by massaging the scalp. Place your fingertips on small areas at a time and use a shampooing movement to move the scalp without letting your fingers slide.

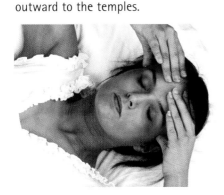

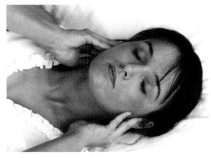

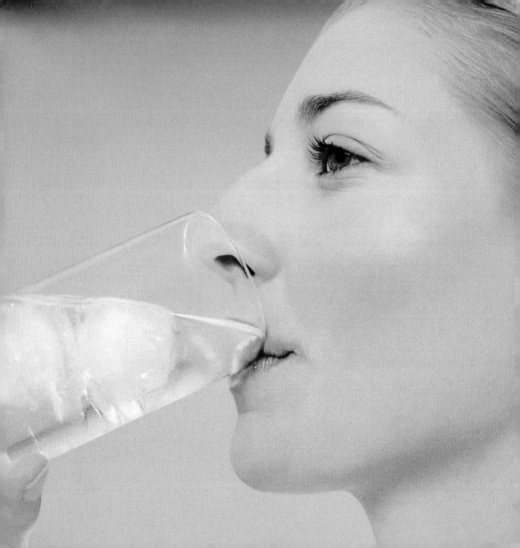

AFTER MASSAGE

A REALLY GOOD MASSAGE TECHNIQUE WILL INVOLVE
SOME SENSITIVITY AFTER THE MASSAGE ITSELF IS COMPLETE.

When you have finished giving a massage, make sure the recipient is warm, comfortable, and well wrapped up. It may well be that they have fallen asleep.

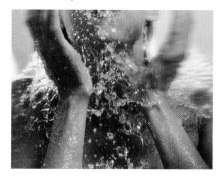

It is a good idea to wash your hands and arms up to the elbows quite vigorously under cold water. Some believe that any negative energy that may have been picked up from the recipient's body by the hands can be released in this way and prevented from entering your body. Regardless of the rationale, you will find this process both refreshing and generally cleansing.

If your recipient is awake, offer them a glass of fresh water. Many people are thirsty after a massage and it is better to avoid stimulants like tea or coffee. Make sure that they are gently brought back to a sense of reality in as calm a manner as possible. If you can, allow the recipient a little time before leaving and try to prevent them from driving too soon afterward. They may not realize just how relaxed they are!

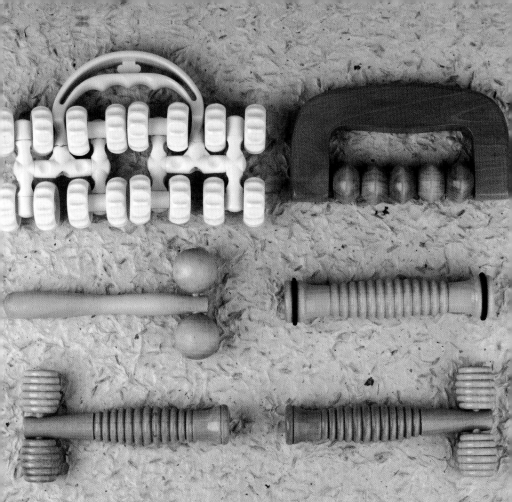

ROLLERS

DIFFERENT ROLLERS FOR MASSAGE CAN BE PURCHASED
READILY AND, WHILE BEING NO SUBSTITUTE FOR HANDS,
THEY CAN BE QUITE BENEFICIAL.

Used for self-massage, rollers can be used to reach places that you can't manage with your hands, especially parts of the back.

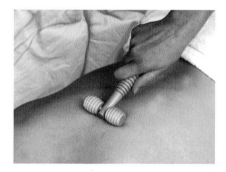

You can also use them on the legs and feet and all fleshy areas of the body. You can even use them while reading, relaxing, or watching television.

Use them carefully when giving someone else a massage and bear in mind it is harder to gauge the pressure you are exerting. Rollers can help to stimulate circulation and the reflex points on the body.

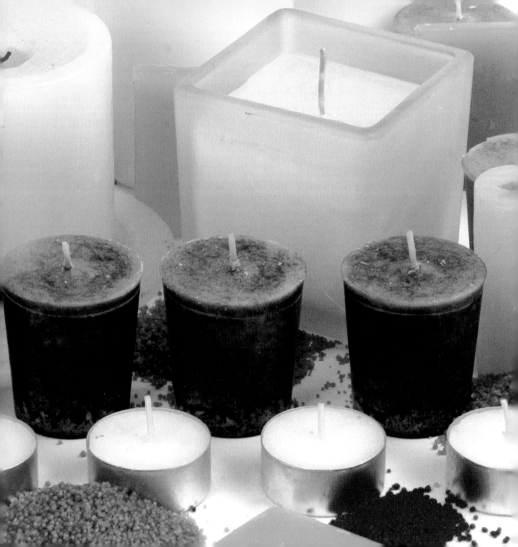

CANDLES

DEPENDING ON WHO YOU ARE MASSAGING, THERE CAN BE
LITTLE TO COMPARE WITH A MASSAGE BY CANDLELIGHT.

Candles give such a warm and
relaxing glow and can only help add
to the benefits of the treatment.
Fragranced candles can help create
an appropriate mood and make the
experience even more pleasant.

Always make sure there is no danger
of them being knocked over. Try using
the apple- and lavender-scented
candles that are included in this
box set.

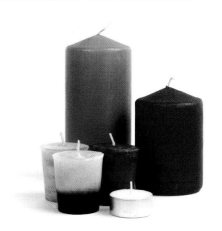

WARNING:

WHILE ALIGHT, ENSURE THAT THE CANDLES ARE
PLACED IN SUITABLE HOLDERS, OR ON AN APPROPRIATE
SURFACE. NEVER LEAVE THEM UNATTENDED AND
KEEP AWAY FROM SOFT FURNISHINGS.
KEEP OUT OF THE REACH OF CHILDREN.

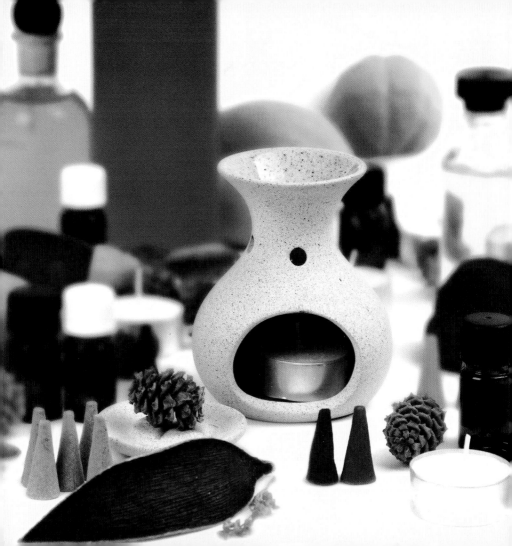

OIL BURNERS

THERE ARE A WIDE VARIETY OF BURNERS COMMERCIALLY AVAILABLE AND THEY ARE TYPICALLY MADE FROM GLASS, METAL, OR CERAMIC MATERIALS.

Oil burners typically consist of a holder for a small candle or tea light, over which sits a container or tray to take water and essential oils.

It is very important that water is used in the container to prevent the oils from heating too rapidly. A few drops of one oil, or a mixture of essential oils, are then added to the water. Most will float on the surface although a few will sink to the bottom.

Light the candle underneath and, as the water heats, the oils will gently warm and evaporate into the room.

They can be very pleasant in a massage room and, as long as they are safely placed, these burners can be a really useful method of dispersing oils and creating the right atmosphere.

Try oils such as marjoram, sandalwood, or tea tree. To freshen a room and lighten the air, any of the citrus oils are wonderful, and because they are antiseptic and bactericidal they will help to cleanse the air as well.

Not only do they get rid of unpleasant smells, they actually kill the bacteria that cause them.

If romance is the order of the day, why not try ylang ylang, rose, or jasmine to help create the right mood?

CONCLUSION

MASSAGE CAN BE THE MOST WONDERFUL THING
BOTH TO GIVE AND RECEIVE.

Massage can be hugely beneficial for the old and young alike, helping to relieve aches and pains and the stresses and strains of everyday life.

It can help bond partners together and be a thoroughly enjoyable shared experience. There must be room in everyone's life for massage at some time.

Do take the time to re-read the sections in this book on Benefits and Safety Tips, and of course, take extra care with frail or elderly people.

If you are attempting to mix your own massage oils, be cautious when adding essential oils. It is better to use less to start with as you can always add more, but you can't take them away once you have put them in. Always carry out a skin test before using a new oil.

Touch is a wonderful thing and massage is a good way to explore this sense. The movements given are only suggestions and a place to start; there is nothing wrong with adapting them to suit yourself. Hopefully they will encourage you to experiment and make up new movements yourself. Most importantly, enjoy rediscovering the benefits of touch.